STOP A[...]

S0-AWQ-048

Here is the breakthrough program that can help eliminate the pain of osteoarthritis forever.

FACT: Two dietary supplements—glucosamine and chondroitin sulfate—can actually reverse the common—and painful—effects of osteoarthritis.

FACT: Antioxidants—such as vitamins A, C, and E—actually prevent further damage to the cartilage and joints.

FACT: Dietary changes can help heal the joint. Eliminating certain foods may help relieve inflammation and pain.

FACT: Painkillers and anti-inflammatory drugs can actually compound osteoarthritis problems.

Let your body heal itself naturally, and join the thousands of people who have already discovered

THE ARTHRITIS SOLUTION

Larry Katzenstein was for six years the medical editor at *American Health* magazine and served for twelve years as a health writer at *Consumer Reports.* He has won national recognition for his medical writing, including the New York Newspaper Guild's Page One Award for Excellence in Journalism/Crusading Journalism Category, and numerous other awards in the field of health.

THE
ARTHRITIS
SOLUTION

Larry Katzenstein

A Lynn Sonberg Book

A SIGNET BOOK

SIGNET
Published by the Penguin Group
Penguin Putnam Inc., 375 Hudson Street, New York, New York 10014, U.S.A.
Penguin Books Ltd, 27 Wrights Lane, London W8 5TZ, England
Penguin Books Australia Ltd, Ringwood, Victoria, Australia
Penguin Books Canada Ltd, 10 Alcorn Avenue,
Toronto, Ontario, Canada M4V 3B2
Penguin Books (N.Z.) Ltd, 182-190 Wairau Road, Auckland 10, New Zealand

Penguin Books Ltd, Registered Offices:
Harmondsworth, Middlesex, England

First published by Signet, an imprint of Dutton Signet,
a member of Penguin Putnam Inc.

First Printing, August, 1997
10 9 8 7 6 5 4 3 2 1

To my wife, Julie, for her patience in putting up with piles of papers, and to my uncle, Dr. John Hassall, for his valuable long-distance assistance in answering my questions about arthritis.

Contents

THE
ARTHRITIS
SOLUTION

Chapter 1

The Arthritis Solution

If you're reading this book, there's a good chance you have osteoarthritis. It is one of the most common health problems in the world, dating back hundreds of thousands of years and affecting most every creature that has ever had joints. It has been found in the fossilized skeleton of the dinosaur Diplodocus, in Neanderthal man, in Egyptian mummies, and in dogs, horses, and other present-day creatures—including some forty million Americans.

Osteoarthritis affects the all-important cartilage that cushions and protects the ends of the bones within the joint. It causes this cartilage to break down, to the point that bone rubs against bone inside the joint—causing the symptoms you're all too familiar with.

The main symptoms of osteoarthritis are pain, stiffness, and joint immobility, and they can make your life an ordeal. These symptoms mean abandoning the recreational activities you most enjoyed, like tennis, golf, or gardening. They mean saying no to the grandchild who wants a piggyback ride or the spouse who wants to go dancing or engage in more intimate romantic activities with you. They mean, ultimately, pulling back from life, shunning the very activities that truly make it worth living.

Not surprisingly, many people with osteoarthritis feel hopeless about their condition and are resigned to watching it get worse as they get older. Adding insult to injury, people with osteoarthritis usually don't get much sympathy from family, friends, or coworkers. They know you're not going to die from the condition, and they view it as merely an inevitable consequence of growing old, something they'll have to contend with eventually as well. Until recently, most doctors shared that dismissive attitude and pretty much ignored osteoarthritis as a field of research. After all, they assumed, here was a condition that's a natural result of wear and tear on the joints, so you can't do much about it except treat the pain that it causes.

Fortunately, that fatalistic stance toward osteoarthritis is now as extinct as the dinosaurs. As you'll learn in *The Arthritis Solution*, you *can* do something about osteoarthritis—now. Two nutritional supplements, chondroitin and glucosamine sulfate, can not only relieve the symptoms but can stop osteoarthritis in its tracks and even help rebuild the all-important joint cartilage that has been lost to the disease.

The strategies outlined in *The Arthritis Solution* are the culmination of more than a decade's worth of research that has led to exciting insights into osteoarthritis. Rather than being some passive disease in which the joints slowly deteriorate, it's now clear that osteoarthritis is actually a dynamic process—a battle royal within the joints where the body's efforts to rebuild damaged cartilage are ultimately overwhelmed by processes that break cartilage down.

The good news is that you can win this battle by

intervening at an early stage, before damage to the joints becomes severe. Simply follow the three-pronged attack described in these pages.

1. *Take glucosamine and chondroitin sulfate supplements.* These two supplements are the most promising advances in decades in the treatment of osteoarthritis. Both are natural components of cartilage. When you take them in supplement form, they act at the cellular level to help cartilage rebuild itself and to protect it from further breaking down. These two dietary supplements can help you turn the tide against cartilage breakdown and restore cartilage to health.

   The proven ability of glucosamine and chondroitin sulfate to help people with osteoarthritis has been overlooked for far too long. Some fifteen clinical studies conducted overseas, mostly in Europe, have found that many osteoarthritis sufferers who take those drugs have experienced impressive improvements in their conditions— less pain and stiffness and greatly increased mobility. Both supplements are vital for maintaining healthy joints; they're available without a prescription and they're extremely safe to use. *The Arthritis Solution* tells you how these and other arthritis-fighting supplements work, where you can get them, and the proper dose for optimal benefits.

2. *Eat the right foods.* Certain foods may aggravate osteoarthritis while other foods may help to ease its symptoms. Our "Eat to Beat Osteoarthritis" program tells you which foods to favor and which to avoid. It also tells you about the foods that are rich in antioxidants, the nutrients that

are showing great promise in warding off several major chronic diseases including osteoarthritis. Finally, this chapter offers advice for overcoming one of the leading causes of osteoarthritis: obesity. If you are overweight, shedding pounds is one of the most effective things you can do to relieve your symptoms—and even protect you from developing osteoarthritis in the first place.

3. *Follow our exercise prescription.* The final prong in the antiarthritis attack is exercise. For many years, patients with osteoarthritis have been advised by their doctors to avoid exercise, on the assumption that it would only make things worse by adding to the wear and tear on the joints. But now we know that exercise is an absolutely necessary therapy for arthritis. In fact, today's arthritis experts consider exercise just as effective as drug treatment for relieving pain and improving mobility in people with the disease. According to recent studies, certain exercises can dramatically improve the health of people with osteoarthritis. We'll tell you what exercises are best for the particular joints that are bothering you and help you plan an exercise program that can also improve your overall health.

Lifting the Gloom

The way osteoarthritis has been treated—or more accurately, not treated—is probably the reason that so many patients feel pessimistic about having the disease. Even recently, treatment of osteoarthritis consisted of little more than prescribing pain relievers to soothe symptoms. The drugs usually prescribed—the nonsteroidal anti-inflammatory drugs, or NSAIDs—have no effect on the disease itself. And as we'll see, these potent drugs often cause serious side effects, such as the gastrointestinal bleeding that proves fatal to thousands of people every year. This book can help you cut back on these dangerous drugs or stop taking them entirely.

Glucosamine and chondroitin sulfate are at the core of *The Arthritis Solution*'s strategy against osteoarthritis. We'll tell you everything you need to know about these supplements, which are revolutionizing the way osteoarthritis is treated, and we'll examine the recent dramatic evidence showing that the antioxidant vitamins C, E, and beta carotene can help stop osteoarthritis from worsening.

We'll also take a look at unconventional treatments such as acupuncture, homeopathy, spas, and the drug DMSO, and tell you which ones are truly useful and which you should avoid. Finally, we'll describe gene therapy and other techniques—some highly experimental, some on the verge of widespread use—that are showing great promise.

As you read *The Arthritis Solution*, you'll see that you no longer have to take your osteoarthritis lying down—that you can take charge of your condition and take actions that not only address its underlying causes but that may actually help to reverse it.

What Is Osteoarthritis?

Arthritis is the nation's leading cause of disability. Most of the seven million Americans disabled by the disease have the type known as osteoarthritis—and so do most arthritics whose pain or immobility becomes so extreme that they must be operated on to receive artificial knee, hip, or other joints.

Osteoarthritis affects the cartilage that covers and cushions the ends of the bones within the joint. This cartilage allows the bones to rub together smoothly when you stand up, grasp a pencil, throw a baseball, or perform any of the flexing, bending, or gripping activities of daily life that the joints make possible. In osteoarthritis, the protective cartilage erodes so that bone rubs against bone, causing pain, inflammation, stiffness, and constricted range of motion. The seriousness of these symptoms can vary widely, from being merely inconvenient to being totally disabling.

The traditional synonyms for osteoarthritis—"degenerative" or "wear-and-tear" arthritis—reflect what people had long assumed about the disease: that it was a normal and inevitable part of getting older. And while it's true that osteoarthritis becomes more prevalent with age, it's also clear that the disease is neither inevitable nor a "normal" aspect of aging. Instead, researchers are uncovering a variety of causes for the disease. Some of them, such as obesity and injuries to the joint, can be corrected in time to prevent the disease; other causes, including genetic abnormalities that may account for many cases, may be correctable in the future, particularly through gene therapy.

What Causes Osteoarthritis?

A number of "risk factors" have been identified as increasing a person's chance of developing osteoarthritis. These risk factors account for a significant portion of osteoarthritis cases. You have it in your power to control several of them, and by doing so, you can reduce your chances of developing osteoarthritis. Here are the most important contributing risk factors:

Injury to the joints. Anyone who suffers an injury to some part of a joint—bone, cartilage, ligament, or tendon—faces an increased risk for eventually developing osteoarthritis in that joint. With some injuries, such as a compound fracture of the ankle, osteoarthritis is almost guaranteed. Professional athletes who've suffered frequent knee injuries are also likely to develop osteoarthritis of the knee after their playing days are over. One study found that more than eighty percent of American football players with a history of a knee injury had evidence of osteoarthritis ten to thirty years after competing.

Repetitive stress on the joints. Some people have jobs that increase the chances that they'll develop osteoarthritis. For example, osteoarthritis of the knee is especially common among miners, dockworkers, and others whose jobs involve regular knee bending and heavy lifting. Farming for a living increases one's risk for osteoarthritis of the hip. The hands of jackhammer operators take a pounding that often leads to osteoarthritis in their finger joints. Similarly, professional boxers develop it in the knuckles at the base of their fingers—a site that's uncommon for osteoarthritis in the general population.

Obesity. Over the years, being overweight puts stress on the joints that eventually damages the cartilage, making obesity a major risk factor for osteoarthritis, particularly of the weight-bearing joints—the knee and, to a lesser extent, the hip. One long-term study that followed women of various weights over thirty-six years found that the heaviest women—those in the upper twenty percent of the group—were more than three times likelier to develop severe knee osteoarthritis than were women in the bottom twenty percent of the group by weight.

The good news is that losing weight can greatly alleviate symptoms and actually prevent the disease—and you don't have to lose that much. A 1992 study found that overweight middle-aged and older women could cut their risk of osteoarthritis of the knee in half by losing eleven pounds over ten years.

Loose joints. When bones in the joint aren't held together tightly, movement can create abnormal pressures on the bones that can damage cartilage. Joint instability is now recognized as an important cause of pain and early morning stiffness that may be felt long before cartilage damage has occurred. The symptoms often occur in young "double-jointed" women whose flexibility makes them especially adept at ballet. As a preventive measure, such people may be advised against activities that could increase their risk of developing premature osteoarthritis.

Genetic factors. It's long been recognized that osteoarthritis tends to run in families. In their search for a possible genetic cause, researchers studied a family with members who developed osteoarthritis at a very early age. In 1990, these researchers reported success in identifying the first "osteoarthritis mutation": a defect in a gene responsible for producing collagen, a protein that is an important component of cartilage. The defective collagen probably weakens the cartilage and causes its premature breakdown.

Since then, several other mutations that are involved in causing osteoarthritis have been identified. Some experts believe that at least one-fourth of all cases of osteoarthritis may result from genetic abnormalities. Currently, several teams of researchers are working to develop gene therapy for osteoarthritis, which would involve correcting the genetic defect or replacing abnormal cells with normal ones.

Being female. Women are much more likely to develop osteoarthritis than men, especially as they get older. The gender differences are most extreme for osteoarthritis of the knee in older people. Among people over sixty-five, women are twice as likely as men to have pain, stiffness, and other symptoms of osteoarthritis of the knee.

Getting older. Age has been called the most powerful risk factor for osteoarthritis. For example, only two percent of people under forty-five have osteoarthritis; the prevalence rises to thirty percent of people between forty-five and sixty-four, and for those sixty-five and over, the disease affects between sixty-three percent and eighty-five percent of people. But getting older does not *inevitably* lead to osteoarthritis. The good news from recent studies is that the normal wear and tear on the joints that occurs with age is different from the changes that occur in osteoarthritis.

When researchers examined joint cartilage from elderly people unaffected by the disease and other people the same age with osteoarthritis, they found some striking differences. The people with osteoarthritis had cartilage that contained more water, presumably making the cartilage softer and more fragile. Their cartilage also contained higher levels of chemicals that degrade cartilage.

But perhaps most significant of all for readers of *The Arthritis Solution*, the cartilage in the osteoarthritis sufferers contained scantier amounts of the key cartilage components called proteoglycans. The supplements recommended in *The Arthritis Solution*—chondroitin sulfate and glucosamine—are vital building blocks for synthesizing proteoglycans in cartilage.

These studies deliver a clear message: By taking chondroitin sulfate and glucosamine, you may be able to rebuild proteoglycans and restore damaged cartilage to health. Even more exciting, these two nutrients may help prevent osteoarthritis by keeping cartilage healthy enough that it won't break down.

It's obvious that people can live to ripe old ages and never develop osteoarthritis. The supplements we recommend in *The Arthritis Solution*, along with our other recommendations on diet and exercise, can help you be among them.

THE NUMBERS TELL THE STORY

Many people with arthritis of any kind don't get much sympathy from family and friends. And all too often they disparage their own condition, regarding it not as a genuine disease but rather an embarrassing sign that they're growing older and creakier. It's high time we abandon those misperceptions about arthritis and appreciate it for what it is: a serious health care problem. Consider these facts about this country's number one cause of disability:

- Because of arthritis, more than seven million Americans have trouble performing everyday activities such as dressing, climbing stairs, or getting in and out of bed.

- Each year, arthritis results in forty-five million visits to physicians, four million hospitalizations, and 185 million days spent in bed.
- Arthritis is more prevalent than either heart disease, cancer, or diabetes. Approximately forty million Americans—more than fifteen percent of the total population—have some form of arthritis, of which osteoarthritis is by far the most common type.
- The number of Americans with arthritis has been growing dramatically—and will rise even faster as the baby boomers begin entering their fifties. Estimates indicate that, by the year 2020, the number of Americans with arthritis will have risen from forty million to sixty million.
- Arthritis is sixty percent more common in women than it is in men. A recent federal survey found that twenty-three percent of all adult American women reported joint problems indicative of arthritis. Nine percent of women aged fifteen to forty-four had the condition, thirty-three percent of women forty-five to sixty-four had the problem, and fifty-six percent of women sixty-five and older were affected.
- Osteoarthritis and other diseases of the joints cost the U.S. $150 billion a year—an amount of money equivalent to 2.5 percent of the yearly gross national product. Of that $150 billion, just under half is attributable to the costs of medical care. The remainder comes from indirect costs due to lost wages.

Chapter 2

Is It Osteoarthritis?

While the two supplements we describe in this book, glucosamine and chondroitin sulfate, have achieved some miraculous results when people with osteoarthritis have taken them, you want to be sure that osteoarthritis really is your problem. If your joint pain isn't caused by osteoarthritis, you may not benefit from these supplements. And learning that your joint pain is due to some other arthritic problem may lead you to the proper treatment for your condition.

Your joints are the places in your body at which two or more bones join. There are several joint types, classified according to the range of movement they allow. Fixed joints, the most rigid of all joints, allow no movement at all. Prime examples are the joints, known as sutures, where the bones of the skull come together. But most joints are "movable," and these movable joints allow all the activities involved in living—walking, bending, lifting, climbing, writing, playing the piano, or throwing a baseball. The "movement" of these joints is generated by skeletal muscles that pull on the bones that form the joint. These movable joints are the ones that are affected by osteoarthritis.

Osteoarthritis refers to just one of about a hundred different diseases included in the category of "arthritis." All these forms of arthritis have several things in common: joint pain, joint swelling, joint stiffness, and a restricted range of motion in the joint.

In addition, in every type of arthritis except one, the joints become inflamed (in fact, the term "arthritis" literally means "inflammation of the joints"). Osteoarthritis is the lone exception. In contrast to all other forms of arthritis, the symptoms of osteoarthritis—while often closely resembling those of other forms of arthritis—are not *caused* by joint inflammation, although inflammation may be present.

When a case of osteoarthritis doesn't have an obvious cause, it's referred to as primary arthritis. Most cases of osteoarthritis fall into this category. But when osteoarthritis can be attributed to something specific—a broken ankle, for example, or an old football injury to your knee—it's called secondary arthritis, meaning that it's secondary to some other event. Of course, things aren't always so simple, and it's now recognized that osteoarthritis can result from the sum total of several factors—for example, an injury combined with being overweight combined with physical inactivity.

In osteoarthritis there is stiffness and pain in the affected joint, and often the joint's movement is restricted. People with osteoarthritis may also notice that their joints make crackling sounds (referred to in medical language as "crepitus") as they move them. The joints that bear the most weight, the knees and the hips, are the most vulnerable to osteoarthritis and are the ones most commonly affected. Other joints that often develop osteoarthritis are those in the hands, the feet, and the spine. In the spine, the joints usually affected are those in the neck and the lower part of the back; osteoarthritis of the hand most often strikes the joints at the base of the thumb and the ends of the fingers; and in the feet, the joint most often affected is the one at the base of the big toe.

A notable feature of osteoarthritis is that the pain tends to worsen toward the end of the day. That distinguishes it from many other types of arthritis, in which pain is consistent throughout the day or worse in the morning. As for the stiffness of osteoarthritis, it usually occurs after you've been inactive for a while. For example, you may notice that your joints have "frozen" or "locked up" when you climb out of the car after a long drive or while you're walking out of the theater after watching a movie. (On the plus side, the stiffness of osteoarthritis usually diminishes several minutes after you've resumed activity and gotten the joints loosened up.)

The Arthritis Checkup

To find out if your symptoms are really caused by osteoarthritis and to rule out more serious conditions, you need to be examined by a doctor. A diagnosis of osteoarthritis is usually based on several things, including the symptoms you have, your history of joint problems, and a physical examination.

During the exam, the doctor will look for the physical signs of osteoarthritis, which include pain in the affected joint, the growth of bony swellings or spurs (known as osteophytes) at the ends of the bones in the affected joint, and mild signs of inflammation (including swelling, redness, or joint tenderness). In addition, the doctor will ask to see how far you can bend the joint, to see if there has been any loss of the joint's normal range of movement.

While you're moving your joint through its range of motion, your doctor will place his or her palm against the joint to feel for that crackling sensation mentioned earlier, which results from damage to the cartilage surfaces. The doctor will also test the joint for stiffness by positioning his or her hands on either side of the joint and gently moving it as far as pain or swelling in the joint may allow. Finally, the doctor may take an X ray to confirm that osteoarthritis is affecting the joint. The X ray signals a diagnosis of osteoarthritis if no space appears between the bones of the joint—a sign that cartilage, which is not visible on an X ray, has worn away and that bone is now pressing on bone.

If your doctor has trouble diagnosing the cause of your joint problem or has failed to help the problem, you should consider asking for a referral to a specialist or finding one on your own. Physicians who specialize in diagnosing and treating osteoarthritis and other forms of arthritis are called rheumatologists. These doctors are internists—specialists in internal medicine—who have taken two additional years of training in the treatment of arthritis and other so-called rheumatic diseases.

There are several ways for you to find a rheumatologist:

- Ask a physician you know or a neighbor or friend to recommend a good rheumatologist.
- Call your local medical society, which should maintain a list of doctors who belong to the various medical specialties.

- Look in the yellow pages under "physicians" and then find the subheading "rheumatology."
- Call your local chapter of the Arthritis Foundation. If you're not able to locate a local chapter, call the organization's national office in Atlanta toll-free at 800-283-7800.
- Contact the rheumatologists' membership organization, the American College of Rheumatology, also in Atlanta, at 404-633-3777.

Exploring the Joint

Before focusing on the joint—the central character in the drama of osteoarthritis—we need to mention those structures that literally play key supporting roles for the joints: the ligaments and tendons.

Ligaments are strong, flexible bands of tissue that attach to bone and bind bones together, including the two bones within a joint. Assisting the ligaments in stabilizing and supporting the joints are the tendons, which attach muscle to bone. When a muscle contracts and "moves" a joint—in a bending finger, for example—the tendon is the intermediary through which the muscle pulls on the bone. As we'll see in Chapter 8, one reason exercise is so important for people with osteoarthritis is that it strengthens the ligaments and tendons—and strong ligaments and tendons move the joints much more easily.

The joint itself is enclosed and protected by a tough, fibrous covering known as the joint capsule. The capsule's outer layer is formed by fibers made of the protein collagen that are arranged in parallel bands surrounding the joint; interlaced with these bands are other collagen fibers. This arrangement of interwoven fibers gives the joint capsule its strength and flexibility.

The tough joint capsule's inner surface is lined with a delicate layer of tissue called the synovial membrane. This membrane contains numerous blood vessels as well as the cells that constantly secrete synovial fluid—the lubricating fluid for the joints. Synovial fluid is ninety-five percent water and is clear, yellowish, and sticky, with a consistency resembling the white of an egg.

The heart of the joint is where the bones meet. At this crucial location, the ends of the bones are covered with a tough, smooth, slippery coating of cartilage known as articular cartilage ("articular" refers to the joints). Aided by the synovial fluid that bathes it, articular cartilage allows a joint to move with even less friction than occurs when ice slides on ice. Articular cartilage has the ability to repair itself in response to normal wear and tear—maintenance work that's done by specialized cartilage cells called chondrocytes, which secrete the tough, fibrous connective tissue that is the basic material of cartilage.

Since cartilage has no blood vessels of its own, its chondrocytes rely on the synovial fluid to provide the nutrients they need to maintain and rebuild cartilage. As we'll see, research has shown that glucosamine and chondroitin sulfate—the dietary supplements that are the focus of *The Arthritis Solution*—pass from the synovial membrane into the synovial fluid and then become incorporated into the cartilage.

These nutrients are two of the key building blocks that the chondrocytes use to make more cartilage. It's when cartilage production can't keep up with cartilage destruction, caused by injury or other factors, that articular cartilage begins wearing away, and the road to osteoarthritis begins. Taking chondroitin sulfate and glucosamine sulfate in supplement form can rebuild cartilage and possibly help reverse osteoarthritis by stimulating the chondrocytes to add more cartilage where it's needed.

How Osteoarthritis Happens

Osteoarthritis usually develops gradually within the joints and does so in a characteristic way. In the early stages, as the articular cartilage starts to break down, the cartilage surfaces become rougher and thinner as they rub against each other. Small chunks of articular cartilage may break off and float around in the synovial fluid, sometimes irritating the synovial membrane—causing the membrane to pump out excess amounts of synovial fluid and making the membrane inflamed, painful, and abnormally thick. At this stage, the joint's range of motion may start to become restricted.

Next, bone spurs made of articular cartilage and bone may form around the outer edge of the joint. Known technically as osteophytes, these painful bone spurs may be the bone's defensive response to the extra pressure it must bear as its cartilage covering wears away. Bone spurs give the joints the knobby, swollen appearance that's particularly apparent in many people who have osteoarthritis of the fingers.

In advanced cases of osteoarthritis, almost all the articular cartilage wears away. No longer able to glide on their cartilage coverings, sensitive bones now rub against each other in the joint. This results in the symptoms of osteoarthritis that are all too familiar: pain, stiffness, and restricted range of motion that can

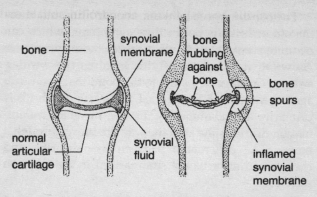

bone

synovial membrane

bone rubbing against bone

bone spurs

normal articular cartilage

synovial fluid

inflamed synovial membrane

**Normal Joint and Joint Affected
by Severe Osteoarthritis**

be virtually paralyzing. Each year, thousands of people with severe osteoarthritis undergo joint replacement operations to relieve their severe pain and regain joint mobility.

Ruling Out Rheumatoid Arthritis

Those key symptoms of osteoarthritis—pain, stiffness, and restricted range of motion—also apply to most of the other numerous forms of arthritis. It's especially important that you know your symptoms stem from osteoarthritis and are not due to rheumatoid arthritis. Unfortunately, the two types of arthritis are often confused—which can lead to serious problems, since the two disorders are managed quite differently. It's important to determine if you do have rheumatoid arthritis, since prompt treatment can slow the devastation of joints that often occurs in this disease.

The big difference between osteoarthritis and rheumatoid arthritis is not in their symptoms, which can be quite similar, but in what causes those symptoms. As we've noted, osteoarthritis involves the wearing away of cartilage in a joint, to the point that bones rub against each other. By contrast, rheumatoid arthritis is primarily an inflammatory disease, in which inflammation destroys the joint the way fire burns through a house. The differences between osteoarthritis and rheumatoid arthritis are summarized in the table on page 21.

A Disease of Inflammation

The inflammation in rheumatoid arthritis is centered on the synovial membrane, the inner lining of the capsule that surrounds the joints. When this membrane becomes inflamed, it causes heat, swelling, stiffness, and pain all around the joint. Over time, this chronic inflammation invades and damages the bone and cartilage of the joints and also spreads to and weakens the surrounding muscles, tendons, and ligaments. Ultimately, the inflammation can destroy the joints and cause loss of movement when the bones that form the joint fuse together.

While both osteoarthritis and rheumatoid arthritis can cause crippling, rheumatoid arthritis is considered the more serious of the two diseases. It usually affects many more of a person's joints than does osteoarthritis, and it is more likely to cause severe damage in the joints that it affects.

Rheumatoid arthritis's inflammation can be traced to an autoimmune reaction, which means that a glitch in the body's immune system causes it to recognize

Osteoarthritis and Rheumatoid Arthritis: The Crucial Differences

Prevalence

Osteoarthritis: Increasingly common with age, affecting up to eighty-five percent of people over sixty-five

Rheumatoid: Affects approximately one percent of the population

Age of Onset

Osteoarthritis: Age forty-five to ninety

Rheumatoid: Children nearing adolescence; adults in their twenties to fifties

Disease Pattern

Osteoarthritis: Rarely affects both joints (e.g., both knees) at once

Rheumatoid: Often strikes symmetrically (e.g., both wrists, both knees)

Joints Affected

Osteoarthritis: Usually the feet, knees, hips, hands, and spine; sometimes the knuckles and wrists; rarely elbows and shoulders

Rheumatoid: Affects many of the joints, including the knuckles, wrists, elbows, and shoulders

Speed of Onset

Osteoarthritis: Develops slowly, usually over several years

Rheumatoid: Develops suddenly, within weeks or months

Extent of Illness

Osteoarthritis: Limited to the joints

Rheumatoid: In addition to joint damage, can cause sickness and fatigue, fever, anemia, and weight loss and attack healthy joint tissue as if it were a foreign invader. It's this attack that causes the inflammation that can severely damage the joints. (Other autoimmune diseases that attack various other parts of the body include juvenile diabetes, lupus, and multiple sclerosis.)

Researchers suspect that some people have inherited a susceptibility to this autoimmune reaction, enabling an event like a viral infection to trigger the autoimmune response that results in rheumatoid arthritis. This theory is supported by the fact that most people who have the disease also have a genetic marker called HLA-DR4, which is a tissue type similar to a blood type. (The good news is that most of the twenty-five percent of the population who have this marker will not develop rheumatoid arthritis.) Women are more susceptible than men to autoimmune diseases, so it's not surprising that, of the 2.5 million American adults who have rheumatoid arthritis, three-fourths are women.

The majority of people with rheumatoid arthritis develop it between the ages of thirty-five and fifty, in contrast to osteoarthritis, which is primarily a disease of older people. Rheumatoid arthritis is characterized by a feeling of general fatigue, stiffness, and achiness. Usually, the joints affected first are in the wrists, fingers, feet, or knees. Additional joints may become painful and swollen as the disease progresses.

A lucky minority of people with symptoms of rheumatoid arthritis—between ten and twenty percent—will recover completely within a few years of developing it. Another five to ten percent of sufferers have acute cases that develop rapidly and cause severe disability. But most commonly, the disease progresses slowly in a cyclical way, with periodic flare-ups of symptoms alternating with months or even years during which symptoms almost disappear. In people with this chronic form, rheumatoid arthritis is often systemic, meaning that inflammatory problems go beyond the joints to affect the nerves, eyes, skin, and blood vessels.

Diagnosing and Treating Rheumatoid Arthritis

The diagnosis of rheumatoid arthritis relies not only on a person's symptoms and the findings of a physical exam but also on two blood tests. One of them tests for rheumatoid factor, which is present in the blood of about eighty percent of adults with rheumatoid arthritis; produced by the immune system, rheumatoid factor is the antibody that contributes to the destructive inflammation in rheumatoid arthritis. Another blood test measures the rate at which red blood cells drop to the bottom of a glass tube; this so-called sedimentation rate, or sed rate, is faster in cases where chronic inflammation is present. In yet another test used in diagnosing rheumatoid arthritis, a needle is used to remove synovial fluid from an affected joint; the presence of white blood cells in the fluid indicates that an inflammatory condition is present.

Not too long ago, total rest was the standard treatment for people with rheumatoid arthritis. But today, most people with rheumatoid arthritis can lead active productive lives, thanks to improvements in drugs and surgical procedures and better insights into managing the disease.

The primary goal in the treatment of rheumatoid arthritis is controlling the destructive inflammation that lies at the root of the disease. Two highly effective types of drugs—the nonsteroidal anti-inflammatory drugs (NSAIDs) and the corticosteroids—have revolutionized the treatment of rheumatoid arthritis by relieving patients' inflammation and pain and improving joint mobility. But both types of drugs can cause serious side effects, and patients being treated with them must be monitored carefully.

Other potent medications, the disease-modifying antirheumatic drugs, are slow-acting drugs that may require several months to produce improvements. Examples include several gold compounds and the drugs penicillamine and chloroquine. Scientists don't yet understand how these drugs work, and they can cause potentially dangerous side effects.

Treatment options other than drugs are also available to people with rheumatoid arthritis. Exercise can keep the joints mobile and improve physical fitness, while rest is generally recommended during a flare-up of symptoms. Physical therapists can help by administering massage and other forms of therapy. In severe cases, surgery can be used to replace immobile or deformed joints.

Other Types of Arthritis

Joints that are painful and stiff are also present in a number of other diseases, which can be confused with osteoarthritis. Some you should know about include the following:

Gout. First described in Hippocrates more than two thousand years ago, this ancient malady was once known as "the disease of kings" since it seemed to be caused by overindulgence in food and drink. And indeed, of all the arthritic diseases, gout is most clearly linked to diet.

Gout attacks can damage the joints, and this disease was once a major cause of painful and crippling chronic arthritis. Fortunately, effective drugs for gout are now available, but all too many of the one million Americans with gout are not aware of that fact.

Attacks of gout occur when excess amounts of uric acid in the blood trigger the formation of needlelike uric acid crystals, which typically accumulate in one of the joints—most commonly the big toe but sometimes the knee or the knuckles. Once inside the joint, these gritty particles can cause excruciating pain and inflammation.

Untreated, gout attacks can last for several days; during that time, the affected joint is hot, inflamed, and highly sensitive to the touch. The attacks usually subside as quickly as they began. Before today's long-term treatments became available, gout sufferers lived in constant fear of their next attack—which might not be for many months or even years. (Without treatment, first-time gout sufferers will have a second attack within a year, and three-fourths can expect a recurrence within four to five years.) Between eighty and ninety percent of gout sufferers are men, who usually experience their first attack between the ages of forty and fifty.

The excess uric acid levels in the blood that give rise to gout can result from too much uric acid being produced by the body or too little of it being eliminated by the kidneys; both of these glitches may be genetic in origin, since gout definitely runs in families. Alternatively—and here is the "disease of kings" connection—these excess uric acid levels can be due to eating too much food rich in purines, chemicals that the body metabolizes into crystal-causing uric acid. One way to avoid gout is by going easy on foods that are high in purines, such as certain meats (liver is particularly rich in purines), seafoods (especially anchovies), as well as dried peas and beans. It's also a good idea to avoid alcoholic beverages, since alcohol can increase uric acid levels.

In addition to watching their diet, people who are prone to gout can take advantage of some highly effective drugs. While no drug can cure gout, some of them can ease the discomfort of gout attacks while others can prevent the attacks from occurring.

Colchicine—a drug used in gout treatment since the 1800s—is effective in treating gout attacks. It relieves the pain and swelling, but it often causes intestinal upset. The nonsteroidal anti-inflammatory drugs are effective and better tolerated, but they also have side effects—particularly the irritation they cause to the gastrointestinal tract. The biggest advance against gout was the development in the 1950s of drugs that prevent gout attacks from occurring by controlling uric acid levels in the blood. These drugs are allopurinol, probenecid, and sulfinpyrazone, and their effectiveness in preventing gout represents one of medicine's most clear-cut victories against any form of arthritis. To be effective, these three drugs must be taken indefinitely.

Pseudogout. Pseudogout is a separate arthritic condition that's similar to gout but involves the presence in the joints of different types of crystals—in this case, calcium pyrophosphate crystals, which usually form for no known reason. Pseudogout most often affects the knees but can also strike the wrists and ankles, and its crystalline deposits can cause severe degeneration of these joints. The disease is very common, especially among older people. It affects about three percent of people in their sixties and becomes ever more common in later decades, striking as many as half of all people over ninety. Treatment is largely limited to treating the pain and disability of pseudogout attacks, usually with nonsteroidal anti-inflammatory drugs or with injections of corticosteroids into the joints.

Fibromyalgia. This somewhat mysterious condition has only recently been recognized as a medical disorder, yet it now ranks as one of the most common types of arthritis, second only to osteoarthritis in prevalence. Its most prominent feature is pain—always present to some degree, usually widespread and sometimes quite severe. For some reason, people with the disorder also seem to be more sensitive to pain than others. Other symptoms can include migraine headache, fatigue, sleep disorders, irritable bowel syndrome, and depression. Anywhere from three to six million Americans are believed to have fibromyalgia, which affects seven times more women than men, particularly women of childbearing age.

Fibromyalgia is mysterious because its cause is unknown, there is no cure (although some treatments are useful in dealing with the symptoms), and it's quite difficult to diagnose. Some patients, in fact, spend years seeking an accurate diagnosis, with doctor after doctor telling them that the problem is "all in their head." More often than not, fibromyalgia is diagnosed by process of elimination, with patients going through batteries of tests to rule out other conditions as the cause of their pain. And even when a diagnosis is made, people with fibromyalgia often look healthy and show no abnormalities on laboratory tests.

One clue that a person has fibromyalgia is the presence of "tender points"—specific areas of tenderness, located in various muscles and bones, that hurt when pressure is applied. Often patients aren't aware of these tender points until a doctor applies pressure to them.

At present, treatment for fibromyalgia is limited to soothing its symptoms. NSAIDs and other pain relievers can help to minimize the pain, and stress reduction, physical exercise, and low doses of antidepressant medication can help promote better sleeping.

Polymyositis. This disease, which literally means "inflammation of many muscles," features generalized muscle weakness that's usually painless. Muscles most commonly affected are those of the shoulders, upper arms, thighs, and hips. Swallowing or lifting the head can be difficult in cases where muscles of the neck and chest are affected. Other symptoms may include fever, weight loss, and joint pain.

Polymyositis is not well understood but is thought to be caused by a malfunctioning immune system. In a recent study, nearly half of all polymyositis patients improved about being treated with oral corticosteroids, which are potent anti-inflammatory drugs. The chance of successful treatment was highest in patients who were treated soon after their disease was diagnosed.

Reiter's syndrome. This is a chronic, intermittent arthritic condition that can also involve inflammation of other parts of the body, particularly the urethra and the eyes, which develop conjunctivitis (inflammation of the membrane covering the white of the eye and lining the inside of the eyelids). The syndrome results from the body's abnormal response to infections elsewhere in the body—either sexually transmitted diseases (STDs) or infections of the gastrointestinal tract. Reiter's syndrome typically affects young men between the ages of twenty and forty who develop it after becoming infected with an STD.

People with this disorder have a genetic susceptibility that has been traced to a particular gene called HLA-B27. When people with this gene are exposed to specific types of bacteria, such as the bacterial species that causes the STD chlamydia, approximately one in five will go on to develop Reiter's syndrome.

The arthritis from Reiter's syndrome usually starts in the knees, feet, or ankles. NSAIDs can help to minimize the pain and inflammation. But if recurrent bouts of the syndrome are to be prevented, the infection causing it must be treated as well.

Bursitis. Bursitis doesn't actually involve the joints, but it's often mistaken for osteoarthritis. It involves inflammation or irritation of a bursa, a small sac filled with synovial fluid that is found near certain joints, including the knee and elbow. A bursa functions as a cushion, helping to prevent the parts of a joint from damaging each other by rubbing together. For example, the infrapatellar bursa, one of several near the knee, prevents wear and tear between the tibia (shinbone) and the tendon that passes over it. When a bursa becomes irritated or inflamed, it fills with excess synovial fluid and swells up, becomes painful, or both. The skin that covers the bursa may feel warm to the touch and look redder than usual.

Bursitis tends to develop when people place a great deal of pressure on a particular joint, such as carpet installers who must kneel for long periods of time ("housemaid's knee") or students who subject their elbows to prolonged pressure while studying at a desk or table ("student's elbow"). In addition, bursitis can result from infections in nearby tissues, a blow or other injury to a joint, or a joint's forceful repetitive movement.

Often the best treatment for bursitis is a few days' rest, which allows the bursa's excess fluid to be reabsorbed into the bloodstream. In addition, ice can help relieve the inflammation, and the pain can be relieved by acetaminophen or a nonprescription dose of an NSAID such as aspirin or ibuprofen (Advil, Nuprin). A bursa that's chronically inflamed may have to be removed through minor surgery. The procedure, called a bursectomy, is usually performed on an outpatient basis unless the swelling is severe or the bursa is infected and the infection seems to be spreading.

Tendinitis. Tendons are crucial to movement: When a muscle contracts, it pulls on its tendon, which in turn pulls on the bone to which it's attached. Tendinitis, the inflammation of a tendon, usually occurs when the outer surface of a tendon rubs against a bone (generally not the bone to which it's attached). The symptoms are pain, tenderness, and, sometimes, restricted movement of the muscle that is attached to the tendon. These symptoms don't always respond to antiinflammatory medications such as the NSAIDs. Other treatments may be needed to reduce inflammation, including ultrasound (use of high-frequency sound waves) and injection of corticosteroid at the site of the inflammation.

Ankylosing spondylitis. Does your back pain become more severe after you've been resting, and does the stiffness in your back and hips sometimes last for hours? If so, you may have ankylosing spondilitis—a disease that in its early stages is often mistaken for a strained back. ("Ankylosing" means stiff, "spondyl" refers to the spine, and "itis" means inflammation.)

Ankylosing spondylitis is mainly a disease of the spine, which becomes inflamed at first, with severe cases resulting in the spinal vertebrae actually becoming fused. Older people who walk hunched over, looking down at the ground, are generally in the late stages of ankylosing spondylitis.

Ankylosing spondylitis typically begins in the sacroiliac joints, which are located in the lower back—on both sides of the spine and just above the buttocks. Later on, the disease moves up to the middle and upper back and often spreads to other joints as well. It's definitely a disease of young people, often beginning before the age of twenty and rarely beginning after forty. Diagnosed three times more frequently in men than in women, ankylosing spondylitis has traditionally been considered a male disease. But research now suggests that men and women may be affected equally, with women usually having much milder cases that usually escape detection.

Ankylosing spondylitis appears to have a genetic cause—specifically, it's confined mainly to people with a defect in a gene called HLA-B27, which plays a role in fighting infections. But the gene defect appears to create susceptibility to the disease rather than actually cause it, since about only twenty percent of people with the defect develop ankylosing spondylitis. Researchers are searching for some other factor—perhaps an environmental toxin or infectious agent—responsible for triggering the disease in susceptible people.

When people with ankylosing spondylitis are diagnosed early, they can usually lead relatively normal lives. The key to treatment is preventing and delaying spinal deformity, which can be accomplished through daily exercises and training in good posture. NSAIDs are usually prescribed to relieve the joint inflammation and pain.

Infectious arthritis. In contrast to most other types of arthritis, which are incurable, infectious arthritis can be cured if the specific infectious organisms responsible for it are effectively treated. Infectious arthritis can be caused by most of the major types of disease-causing microbes—viruses, bacteria, and fungi. Typically, the infectious agent first causes some other health problem and then, after getting established in the body, spreads to the joints and causes arthritis.

The best-known example of infectious arthritis is Lyme disease. It was first identified in 1975, after thirty-nine children and twelve adults living near Lyme, Connecticut, were involved in a mysterious outbreak of crippling arthritis. Lyme disease is caused by a type of bacteria called a spirochete, which is transmitted by the deer tick. People get infected when spirochete-infected ticks attach themselves to the skin and start sucking blood, propelling spirochetes from the tick into the person's bloodstream.

Lyme disease is now the country's most common tick-borne ailment, with more than fifty thousand cases diagnosed since the disease was first discovered. It usually occurs in two distinct stages, early and chronic Lyme disease. The first sign of infection is usually a round red rash, resembling a bull's-eye, at the site of the bite. As the rash slowly fades away over several weeks, an infected person may come down with a flulike illness, with fever, nausea, chills, aching muscles, and swollen glands. These symptoms are usually short-lived, disappearing in about a week.

At this early stage, Lyme disease can readily be cured by treating for twenty-one days with antibiotics such as tetracycline. But in people who aren't treated, the disease usually progresses to the more serious chronic stage. The most common complication of chronic Lyme disease is arthritis, which affects about sixty percent of sufferers; neurological problems such as memory loss affect fifteen percent and cardiac abnormalities such as irregular heartbeat affect about eight percent of people with chronic Lyme disease. The symptoms of chronic Lyme disease may not appear for months or even years after a tick bite and almost always strike people who have not been treated for the early symptoms. It's not clear whether these later complications are due to an ongoing, active infection or from an autoimmune attack triggered by the original infection.

Although Lyme disease has been reported in almost every state, cases are concentrated in three major areas: along the East Coast from Virginia to Maine, in the upper Midwest, and from northern California to southern Oregon. If you live in these areas and notice that you or someone in your family develops persistent pain in the knees, ankles, or other joints, consider the possibility that Lyme disease may be the cause. Fortunately, two promising vaccines for preventing Lyme disease are now in clinical trials and may be on the market in the next year or two.

Carpal tunnel syndrome. This wrist disorder affects people who keep their wrists in a flexed position for long periods of time. It's primarily known as an occupational hazard affecting keyboard operators, truck drivers, or professional pianists. But it can also affect hobbyists such as tennis players, canoeists, golfers, or needlework enthusiasts. The problem can also crop up during pregnancy, due to fluid changes in the body.

The chronic wrist flexing presses on and irritates the median nerve in the hand, causing the nerve to become inflamed at the point where it passes between the bones and a ligament at the front of the wrist. The result is numbness, tingling, and pain in the hand and sometimes the forearm as well. The pain may be especially severe at night.

If possible, the best treatment for carpal tunnel syndrom is to stop doing whatever activity requires you to flex your wrist. The nerve inflammation may also subside with the use of a splint that immobilizes the wrist and thereby minimizes pressure on the nerve. Local injections of cortisone can also reduce the swelling and pain.

People who aren't helped by these options may opt for surgery to relieve their carpal tunnel distress. The operation is relatively simple and can be performed as an outpatient procedure under local anesthesia. The surgical procedure, called carpal tunnel release, involves cutting the ligament in the wrist to relieve pressure on the nearby median nerve. After the operation, patients must wear a supporting wrist splint for a while and do special exercises to restore flexibility to the fingers and wrists.

Raynaud's disease. This circulatory disorder often accompanies other types of arthritis, including rheumatoid arthritis. In Raynaud's disease, spasms occur in the blood vessels of the fingers and toes, causing them to change color—first white, then purple or blue, and finally red—and sometimes become numb. These changes are usually triggered by exposure to cold or emotional stress.

People susceptible to Raynaud's disease should be especially careful about staying warm in cold weather by wearing multiple layers of clothing. Drugs known as calcium channel blockers, which are mainly used for treating high blood pressure, can also help in treating Raynaud's syndrome.

Once your doctor has ruled out these other possible cause of your joint pain, it's quite likely that your problem is osteoarthritis, the most common of all forms of arthritis. In the chapters that follow, we provide the latest information—on drugs, dietary supplements, diet, and exercise—that can help you to minimize the pain and disability that osteoarthritis can cause.

Chapter 3

Arthritis Drugs—Some Benefits, Many Risks, No Cures

If you've been diagnosed with osteoarthritis, you've already heard the bad news about what you can expect. "This is a progressive disease," your doctor has probably told you. "As time goes on, I'll be prescribing increasingly powerful drugs with some nasty side effects, and hopefully they'll be able to control the pain as your joints continue to deteriorate. But there may well come a point when even the strongest drugs can't do the job, and then I'll have to recommend surgery to fit you with artificial joints."

You probably *won't* hear the news that millions of Americans suffering from osteoarthritis need to hear: that you don't have to sit by while your disease turns you into a pain relief junkie or the Six Million Dollar Man. As we'll see, nonpharmaceutical alternatives have been proven to work just as well as drugs in relieving pain and can actually keep the disease from worsening.

You can get substantial pain relief from exercise and from what you eat and don't eat. Even simple measures like applying cold and heat are surprisingly effective. But the most exciting alternative to drugs—the one that may wean you off them once and for all—is the one-two combination of two dietary supplements, glucosamine and chondroitin sulfate. Their ability to relieve pain has been conclusively proven in some fifteen clinical studies. Even more important, these supplements actually alter the disease process at the cellular level rather than merely numb you against the pain.

Drugs "work" against osteoarthritis, but only as Band-Aids that relieve symptoms. Not a single drug can do what's most desperately needed: actually affect what's going on inside the joints—the wearing away of cartilage until bone rubs against bone. By contrast, glucosamine and chondroitin sulfate turn back the pain by working at the cellular level to rebuild and restore damaged and lost cartilage.

After taking glucosamine and chondroitin sulfate for just a few weeks, you can expect to reduce your need for drugs and may ultimately be able to avoid them entirely. That's a worthy goal, because osteoarthritis drugs are a bargain with the devil: People get pain relief in exchange for toxic side effects that kill thousands every year. If you're now taking these drugs, you need to know about their dangers—at least until glucosamine and chonodroitin sulfate will let you evict them from your medicine cabinet.

Anxiety Over NSAIDs

If you're taking a drug for your osteoarthritis pain, chances are it's one of a number of nonsteroidal anti-inflammatory drugs, or NSAIDs (pronounced "en-saids"), which relieve inflammation as well as pain.

For decades, doctors have been treating osteoarthritis patients with these drugs. Aspirin is an NSAID and so are diclofenac, piroxicam, sulindac, and about a dozen other drugs, most available only by prescription. Each year, more than sixty million prescriptions are written for NSAIDs and more than fifteen million patients are receiving long-term therapy with these drugs.

In addition, some of these NSAIDs are now marketed in lower, nonprescription strengths as well. Ibuprofen, for example, is sold by prescription as Motrin and over the counter as Advil, Nuprin, and other brands. (The prescription-strength dosages of these drugs relieve both inflammation and pain, while the lower, nonprescription dosages work against pain but not inflammation.)

Inflammation causes much of the joint damage in rheumatoid arthritis, a rare and often disabling form of arthritis that usually responds well to NSAID therapy. Assuming that inflammation was also behind the pain and stiffness of osteoarthritis, doctors have routinely prescribed NSAIDs for osteoarthritis as well, most commonly diclofenac (Voltaren), naproxen (Naprosyn), and piroxicam (Feldene). But NSAIDs have some major drawbacks. At least one of them, indomethacin (Indocin) actually dissolves cartilage—the last thing you want if you have osteoarthritis. And all of them can cause serious stomach irritation that can sometimes be fatal.

At any given time, about one-fifth of patients receiving long-term NSAID therapy have ulcers—erosions of the lining of the stomach—that can cause serious bleeding or actually perforate the stomach. These gastrointestinal complications from NSAID therapy lead to 76,000 hospitalizations and 7,600 deaths each year in the U.S. Such problems are most likely to affect people who take an NSAID regularly for their arthritis or some other condition; the elderly are at particular risk. These major complications can occur at any time during NSAID treatment, without prior symptoms or any other sort of warning. Long-term users of NSAIDs also face an increased risk of liver disease, kidney disease, and possibly hypertension. Ironically, these serious problems arise from the way the NSAIDs relieve pain and inflammation.

Aspirin and the rest of the NSAIDs all work in the same way: by inhibiting prostaglandins, hormone-like chemicals that are involved in causing pain and inflammation. But unfortunately, the NSAIDs don't discriminate. They not only shut off the "bad" prostaglandins that cause inflammation but also the "good" prostaglandins that form the mucus coating that protects the stomach lining against stomach acid's corrosive effects. The result can be serious stomach bleeding as well as the more common NSAID side effects such as heartburn, upset stomach, indigestion, diarrhea, or constipation.

If you must take an NSAID for your osteoarthritis pain, don't drink alcohol at the same time. Alcohol teams up with the NSAID in your stomach to greatly increase the risk of gastrointestinal irritation. The FDA recently required that labels on all nonprescription pain relievers warn users against taking the drugs if they've consumed three or more drinks that day.

Aspirin, the First Pain Reliever

Ever since it was first sold in the U.S. in 1899, aspirin has been a marketing success story. Aspirin has remained popular for nearly a century for two simple reasons: It works, and it's one of the least expensive drugs around. Two 325-milligram tablets taken at four-hour intervals will relieve mild to moderate pain and reduce fever. (In addition, aspirin exerts an anti-inflammatory effect, which has made it a first-line drug in treating rheumatoid arthritis. Keep in mind that the doses of aspirin necessary to reduce inflammation are well above the maximum levels recommended for relieving minor aches and pains.)

Aspirin works in the same basic way as all NSAIDs do: by inhibiting the prostaglandins that cause pain and inflammation. And as with the other NSAIDs, aspirin can irritate the stomach, since it also knocks out the helpful prostaglandins that protect the stomach lining from being eaten away by acid. But aspirin directly irritates the stomach as well, which makes it the NSAID most likely to cause gastrointestinal problems.

Somewhere between two and ten percent of people who take aspirin even occasionally experience stomach problems, most commonly mild stomach upset or nausea. Heavy users of aspirin, including people who take it regularly and in high doses, face a considerably increased risk of serious bleeding from gastrointestinal ulceration and inflammation. Anyone with stomach ulcers or other gastrointestinal problems should avoid taking aspirin, except under a physician's supervision.

If you take aspirin for your osteoarthritis, there are several different versions available that may help you avoid its irritating impact on the stomach:

Enteric-coated aspirin has a special coating that prevents it from dissolving until it reaches the small intestine. The downside of enteric aspirin is that it's slow to dissolve and therefore takes twice as long to provide pain relief, but it can benefit arthritis patients who take it daily in high doses.

Bufferin and other buffered aspirin products may benefit some people who experience stomach irritation from standard aspirin. Several years ago, researchers tested Bufferin against aspirin and found that, during a three-day study, people taking Bufferin reported one-third fewer stomach reactions than those taking plain aspirin.

Timed-release aspirin tablets typically contain twice the normal dose of aspirin, which is released over a period of six to eight hours. These tablets are not useful for relieving pain or fever, since rapid relief of these symptoms depends on rapid absorption. Timed-release aspirin is marketed mainly to people with arthritis—particularly rheumatoid arthritis—who must maintain an elevated, steady aspirin level in the blood to obtain aspirin's anti-inflammatory effect. This effect has made aspirin valuable for treating rheumatoid arthritis and other disorders in which inflammation plays a central role in causing tissue damage.

Is Aspirin for You?

Aspirin has been around for nearly a century and is still widely used as a pain reliever and for conditions requiring an anti-inflammatory drug. But it causes quite a variety of adverse effects, and sizable numbers of people should avoid it, including anyone who:

- has ulcers, because aspirin can make existing ulcers worse
- is sensitive or allergic to it, as evidenced by a skin rash or shortness of breath after taking it

- has asthma, because it can cause attacks in some asthmatics
- has bleeding disorders or is taking anticoagulant drugs, because aspirin interferes with blood clotting
- has uncontrolled blood pressure, because aspirin increases the risk of stroke in such people
- has liver or kidney disease, because it may make these problems worse
- is a child or adolescent with the flu or chicken pox, because aspirin may cause them to develop Reye's syndrome, a rare but potentially fatal disorder

Over the Counter with Nuprin and Advil

Until 1984, aspirin was the only NSAID available without a prescription. But that year the FDA created front-page news when it approved two new pain relievers, Advil and Nuprin, that contained ibuprofen, a pain-relief ingredient previously available only by prescription. Since then, several other brands of nonprescription ibuprofen have become available, including Medipren, Haltran, Motrin IB, and Midol 200; all of the nonprescription versions contain 200 milligrams of ibuprofen per tablet or caplet. Ibuprofen is a better pain reliever than aspirin and also milder to the stomach. (Motrin, the leading prescription-strength brand of ibuprofen, comes in strengths ranging from 300 to 800 milligrams per tablet.)

In 1994, naproxen joined ibuprofen to become the second previously prescription-only NSAID to make the switch to nonprescription status. So far, just one brand is available—Aleve. When it comes to pain relief, there's no difference between Aleve and nonprescription versions of ibuprofen (Advil, Nuprin, and others). Aleve, however, does have one possible advantage over its ibuprofen competitors: a longer duration of action.

A nonprescription dose of ibuprofen (as well as aspirin and acetaminophen) will work for about four to six hours, after which you can take another dose if you need it. Naproxen, on the other hand, continues to act for up to seven or eight hours in most people, and sometimes even longer. But this longer duration of action can have a downside, since it may increase the risk for NSAID complications such as bleeding or liver or kidney damage. Frequent doses of long-acting Aleve could pose a particular risk to the elderly, since people metabolize drugs less efficiently as they get older. For this reason, Aleve is the only nonprescription pain reliever with a dosage restriction for people over age sixty-five; they're advised not to take the drug more often than once every twelve hours.

The most recent NSAID to make the switch from prescription-only to nonprescription was ketoprofen, which became available in 1995. Two nonprescription brands of ketoprofen are now available, Actron and Orudis KT. Unfortunately, ketoprofen's most notable quality may be its harshness to the gastrointestinal tract. A recent analysis of twelve studies of NSAIDs indicates that Actron and Orudis KT are much more likely to cause stomach upset and intestinal bleeding than any other nonprescription NSAID—even more so than aspirin. The analysis found that ketoprofen is twice as irritating as naproxen (Aleve), more than two and a half times as harsh as aspirin, and four times as harsh as ibuprofen (Advil, Nuprin).

The recommended doses of nonprescription-strength NSAIDs can relieve pain but don't have an anti-inflammatory effect. You need a prescription-strength dose of these NSAIDs to reduce inflammation, but you should never put yourself on a prescription-strength regimen of these drugs without consulting your doctor.

Opt for Acetaminophen

If you need drugs to relieve the pain from osteoarthritis, your best choice may be the nonprescription pain reliever acetaminophen. Sold mainly as Tylenol, acetaminophen was introduced in 1955 and is now the nation's leading pain reliever.

Acetaminophen is quite effective—equal to aspirin and nearly as potent in relieving pain as ibuprofen, naprosyn, and other NSAIDs. Its most distinctive feature is its safety: Considering the millions of doses consumed every year, the drug causes remarkably few side effects.

Acetaminophen's one drawback is that it can't relieve inflammation since it doesn't affect prostaglandins—but that means acetaminophen won't cause the nasty side effects associated with the NSAIDs, either. And if you have osteoarthritis, inflammation probably isn't a problem to begin with.

Inflammation is the main cause of the pain and joint damage in *rheumatoid* arthritis, but experts now believe it plays only a minor role in osteoarthritis. A clinical study published in the *New England Journal of Medicine* in 1991 bolstered that notion and helped make acetaminophen a mainstay of osteoarthritis treatment.

The study involved 184 patients with chronic, persistent knee pain due to osteoarthritis and showed that acetaminophen could work as well against osteoarthritis as prescription-strength NSAID drugs. And if it could do that without posing a risk for the serious side effects associated with regular use of NSAIDs, then it made much more sense to recommend acetaminophen to patients with osteoarthritis. In recent years, other studies have added to the evidence that many people with osteoarthritis don't need NSAIDs for pain relief—even in cases where their joints are actually inflamed.

So in 1995, the American College of Rheumatology made a major change in its guidelines for the management of osteoarthritis. The college recommended that acetaminophen at doses up to 4,000 milligrams per day should be "the initial drug of choice" for treating osteoarthritis of the knee and hip.

As safe as it is, even acetaminophen has been known to cause serious illness and even death. Regular acetaminophen users—those who take it daily over many years—face an increased risk of liver damage as well as kidney damage. But for the most part, problems with acetaminophen almost always result from taking too much of the drug, in amounts far above the maximum recommended dose of 4,000 milligrams per day.

Large overdoses of acetaminophen can cause permanent liver damage or even death. And be careful about taking acetaminophen if you've been drinking alcohol, since serious liver damage can occur if you take excess amounts of acetaminophen during a period of heavy alcohol consumption. Alcoholics face the greatest risk of liver damage from taking high amounts of acetaminophen; older people and those with preexisting liver problems also risk liver damage.

You should also be wary of acetaminophen if you're in the habit of fasting. A 1994 study in the *Journal of the American Medical Association* found that when people who've been fasting consume "moderate overdoses" of acetaminophen—between 4 grams (the maximum amount recommended) and 10 grams per day—they risk liver damage.

The table below lists the various nonprescription pain relievers and also summarizes their main advantages and disadvantages.

PAIN RELIEVERS AT A GLANCE

Acetaminophen

POPULAR BRANDS Tylenol, Anacin-3, Panadol

ADVANTAGES The pain reliever least likely to cause stomach irritation or other unpleasant side effects; especially good for people who have ulcers or are allergic to aspirin; can be used by patients taking blood-thinning drugs since it doesn't interfere with blood clotting; relatively inexpensive (only aspirin is cheaper)

DISADVANTAGES Not an anti-inflammatory drug, so not as effective as the NSAIDs against inflammatory problems such as rheumatoid arthritis and muscle strains; can cause liver damage if excess doses are taken during periods of heavy alcohol consumption; chronic, daily users face an increased risk of liver or kidney damage

Aspirin

POPULAR BRANDS Bayer, Anacin, Bufferin

ADVANTAGES The least expensive of all pain relievers

DISADVANTAGES One of the pain relievers most likely to cause stomach irritation and other potentially serious complications, especially if high doses are taken daily;

less effective than the other NSAIDs as a pain reliever; when taken by children or adolescents with the flu or chickenpox, may cause Reye's syndrome, a potentially fatal illness

Ibuprofen
POPULAR BRANDS Advil, Nuprin, Motrin IB
ADVANTAGES More potent than acetaminophen or aspirin as a pain reliever; equal to the other NSAIDs in pain-relieving ability while least likely of all the NSAIDs to cause complications
DISADVANTAGES May cause irritation and bleeding of the gastrointestinal tract, liver damage, or kidney damage

Naproxen sodium
POPULAR BRANDS Aleve
ADVANTAGES Equal to ibuprofen in effectiveness; doses last longer than other nonprescription pain relievers, so may be useful for pain relief throughout the night (e.g., one dose provides eight to twelve hours of pain relief versus four to six hours for ibuprofen)
DISADVANTAGES Longer-acting doses may increase the risk for complications that NSAIDs typically cause (gastrointestinal tract irritation and bleeding, liver damage or kidney damage), especially for people over sixty-five

Ketoprofen
POPULAR BRANDS Actron and Orudis KT
ADVANTAGES May be faster-acting (noticeable pain relief in thirty minutes) than other pain relievers (forty-five to sixty minutes); equal to ibuprofen in effectiveness
DISADVANTAGES The nonprescription NSAID most likely to cause gastrointestinal tract irritation and bleeding and may also cause kidney or liver damage

A Way to Soothe Irritation?

If—like many people with osteoarthritis—you're a regular NSAID user, you may think that you can prevent NSAID side effects by also taking antacids such as Maalox or Mylanta or acid inhibitors such as Tagamet or Zantac. But that's probably not a good idea. Since they suppress irritation and other symptoms, antacids and similar drugs can cause delays in the detection and treatment of life-threatening bleeding that can occur with NSAID use. There is, however, a prescription drug that may fit the bill. Misoprostol (Cytotec) is the only drug specifically approved by the FDA for preventing the stomach irritation caused by NSAIDs.

As described above, NSAIDs irritate the stomach because they shut down the stomach's production of prostaglandins, which help protect the stomach lining from the acids that continually bathe it. Misoprostol is a synthetic prostaglandin that, when swallowed, helps replace the prostaglandins that are lost due to the action of the NSAIDs. For people whose NSAID intake puts them at high risk for serious stomach irritation—particularly elderly people who must take NSAIDs regularly—misoprostol seems to be quite useful. A recent study of older arthritis patients taking NSAIDs found that misoprostol reduced serious gastrointestinal complications by forty percent.

Two cautions about misoprostol: The drug can cause its own adverse side effects, including diarrhea and cramping. And it may trigger labor if taken by a pregnant woman. The reason: Prostaglandins not only cause pain and inflammation and protect the stomach lining, they also induce uterine contractions—and, in fact, are sometimes purposely administered to induce labor. For this reason, women of childbearing age are urged to use effective contraceptive measures while taking misoprostol and should never begin treatment with misoprostol unless they're absolutely positive that they're not pregnant.

Corticosteroids: Worth the Risk?

NSAIDs aren't the only drugs that can wreak havoc on people with arthritis. Other dangerous but widely used treatments are the corticosteroid drugs, which are used to treat more than thirty million Americans with chronic inflammatory diseases such as asthma, multiple sclerosis, and rheumatoid arthritis. Corticosteroids can dramatically reduce inflammation, but people who take them regularly face enormous risks— most notably, the major bone loss from these drugs that can result in the bone-thinning disorder osteoporosis. Of the twenty million Americans with osteoporosis, an estimated twenty percent—four million people—have it because of their corticosteroid use. Other problems resulting from long-term use of corticosteroids include cataracts, depression, diabetes, and high blood pressure.

You should never take oral corticosteroids for your osteoarthritis. But what about having the drugs injected directly into a painful joint? That can reduce but not prevent the risk of complications and may be helpful—but should be done only occasionally. In three clinical trials involving patients with osteoarthritis of the knee, researchers injected some of the patients with corticosteroids and others with a saline solution. In all three studies, patients whose knees were injected with the corticosteroid felt somewhat better than patients injected with the saline. However, the beneficial effects were not long-lived and after four weeks were no longer apparent.

Doctors caution that the modest and temporary benefits of corticosteroid injections should be weighed against the possible harm they can cause. For one thing, these injections can cause infections inside the joint that can destroy the joint if they are not adequately treated. And injecting corticosteroids frequently into the same joint can eat away the cartilage. For this reason, injections into the same joint should be spaced at least four to six months apart.

Rubbing Away Pain

Rather than being swallowed or injected, some arthritis drugs are rubbed on the body. Such topical drugs that are rubbed on aching joints are technically known as rubefacients, and they may provide noticeable pain relief.

Probably the most effective of these topical pain relievers are the ones containing capsaicin, the chemical that's responsible for the hotness of cayenne and chili peppers. Capsaicin offers temporary pain relief by depleting substance P, a neurotransmitter that carries pain impulses to the brain.

Several well-designed studies involving people with osteoarthritis suggest that capsaicin creams might be worth a try. In one of these studies, people who applied a capsaicin-containing cream to affected joints four times a day for a month obtained significantly more relief of symptoms than those who applied a dummy cream containing no capsaicin.

The relief from capsaicin isn't immediate but usually begins within two to four weeks after treatment starts. For optimal pain relief from capsaicin products, you must apply them frequently, about three or four times a day. As their main adverse effect, capsaicin creams cause a localized burning sensation in about half of users, but this sensation usually decreases the longer the product is used. They're also relatively expensive, especially when used to cover large joints such as the hips. The leading capsaicin products are the creams Zostrix (.025 percent capsaicin) and Zostrix-HP (.075 percent capsaicin), and Dolorac (.25 percent capsaicin); all three are available without a prescription.

You're probably more familiar with other over-the-counter rubefacients, such as Aspercreme and Ben-Gay, which contain salicylates—a family of drugs that reduce pain and inflammation and that include acetylsalicylic acid, the active ingredient in aspirin. Aspirin is certainly an effective pain reliever, but it's less clear that rubbing on salicylate-containing products does much good. At any rate, the salicylate products are not considered as effective as the capsaicin creams. If they do work, it may be because their active ingredients pass through the skin and into the bloodstream—which amounts to a very expensive way of taking aspirin.

In one study, people were asked to rub a methyl salicylate product on a large joint four times a day. Researchers measuring how much of the drug was absorbed into the bloodstream found an amount equal to two aspirin tablets. (Since salicylates can be absorbed, people who are allergic to aspirin should talk with their doctor before using a product that contains it.)

When using any topical pain reliever, always wash your hands after applying them, and make sure the products don't come in contact with easily irritated parts of your body such as your eyes or the mucous membranes lining your mouth or nose.

Pain Relief Recommendations

For the safest possible pain relief for osteoarthritis, choose the dietary supplements glucosamine and chondroitin sulfate (see next chapter). They don't just cover up the pain but instead provide relief by restoring protective cartilage that has been lost. But don't lower your dose of osteoarthritis medication or stop taking it without first consulting your doctor.

If you must take drugs for your osteoarthritis, acetaminophen should be your first choice as a pain reliever. It's much safer and better tolerated than aspirin, ibuprofen, or any of the other NSAIDs and is less expensive than any of the NSAIDs except for aspirin. You can save even more money if you buy generic versions of acetaminophen. The generics are virtually identical to Tylenol and should work just as well.

Use prescription-strength NSAIDs only if you have severely inflamed joints or haven't gotten relief from acetaminophen or from nonprescription NSAIDs such as Advil or Nuprin. According to several recent studies, a significant percentage of patients who are being treated with long-term NSAID therapy could find adequate relief with drugs that are less likely to cause harmful side effects, such as acetaminophen or acetaminophen plus codeine.

If you must use a prescription-strength NSAID to control your symptoms, be aware that none has been found to be consistently better than any other at treating osteoarthritis. Your first choice of an NSAID should probably be ibuprofen, for several reasons. Ibuprofen seems to work as well as other NSAIDs in treating osteoarthritis; it's less expensive than most; and studies have found that ibuprofen produces a lower incidence of serious gastrointestinal side effects than other NSAIDs.

Try to get by with the lowest dose of medication that will control your pain, stiffness, or other symptoms. With NSAIDs—or any drug, for that matter— the higher the dose, the greater the likelihood that you'll experience an adverse effect.

Don't take aspirin and acetaminophen together or capsules containing combinations of the two. In 1995, the National Kidney Foundation warned that aspirin and acetaminophen taken together "increase each other's toxicity and harmful effects on the kidney" and urged that products containing combinations of the two be taken off the market. Examples of such products include Excedrin Extra-Strength and Vanquish.

When taking any pain reliever, you can reduce the risk of stomach irritation by taking it with a full glass of water or shortly after a meal.

If you're really concerned about avoiding stomach upset, stay away from pain relievers such as Anacin and Excedrin that contain caffeine. The caffeine seems to boost the pain relief these products provide, but it can also irritate the stomach.

The American College of Rheumatology recommends that people with osteoarthritis steer clear of one NSAID in particular—the prescription drug indomethacin (Indocin). Evidence indicates that prolonged use of indomethacin may destroy cartilage.

Questions to Ask Before Taking Drugs

So your doctor has recommended that you take a drug or has written you a prescription for one. For your peace of mind and possibly for your own safety, you should ask your doctor or pharmacist some questions before getting that prescription filled. Here are some of the most important questions that need answers:

- How long will it take before this medication starts to work?
- What are the results I should expect and how long should I expect them to last?
- What are the possible side effects from this medication?
- If I start to feel better, can I cut back on the dosage?
- Is this drug available in less expensive generic form?
- Is the drug habit-forming?
- How many times can I get this prescription refilled, if necessary?
- Should I take the medication on an empty stomach or with a meal?
- Are there any foods I should avoid when I take this drug?
- Can this drug interfere with other medications I'm taking, including nonprescription drugs—or can those drugs interfere with my arthritis medication?

Once you've gotten your prescription filled, there are things you can do to ensure that your treatment is safe and effective:

- Always carry with you a list of all the drugs you're taking—both for handy reference and for medical emergencies, when that knowledge can be a tremendous help in determining your problem and giving proper treatment. For example, if you're rushed to the hospital because of severe gastrointestinal bleeding, a doctor who knows that you're taking an NSAID for your arthritis will properly suspect that the drug may be the cause of the bleeding.

- At every visit with your doctor, review any medications you're taking for your osteoarthritis and the proper way to take them.

- Many people with osteoarthritis have other health problems as well. If you consult with more than one doctor, give each of them a rundown on all the drugs you're taking. So if your family doctor prescribes a drug for your hypertension, for example, ask the rheumatologist if that drug could interfere with medications that you're taking for your osteoarthritis.

- A good way to avoid possible drug interactions is to buy all of your drugs at the same pharmacy. Today, many pharmacies use computers to keep track of patients' medications, and some of the computers are programmed to alert the pharmacist when someone has been prescribed drugs that may have unfavorable interactions.

- Don't stop taking a drug or otherwise change your treatment regimen without first consulting your doctor. With any kind of drug, it's tempting to cut back or stop taking it when you start to feel better—which may not be a wise idea. On the other hand, you may feel discouraged if you've been taking a drug for a while without any improvement and be tempted to increase the dosage. But some drugs—especially the NSAIDs that are commonly prescribed for osteoarthritis—may take several weeks of treatment before the benefits kick in.

- Tell your doctor about any changes in your condition since your previous visit, even if you think they have nothing to do with your osteoarthritis or its treatment.
- If you don't understand the explanations or recommendations your doctor gives you, don't feel stupid—speak up and ask for clarification! Expressing things clearly may not be your doctor's strong point.
- Don't be hesitant about discussing your concerns with your doctor, no matter how unimportant you think they are. If something is bothering you, then it definitely isn't trivial.

ARTIFICIAL JOINTS: A MAJOR ADVANCE

It's not always appreciated that osteoarthritis can be an extremely painful disease that destroys joints and cripples people. For people with the most severe cases of osteoarthritis, replacement joints can offer miraculous improvement.

Artificial joints, especially total hip and knee replacements, have revolutionized the treatment of severe osteoarthritis and other types of arthritis. Recipients of hips, knees, and other joints can look forward to virtually painless, much freer joint movement for a decade or more, until the artificial joint needs to be replaced.

Until recently, artificial joints were usually cemented

in place inside the bones. But cemented joints tend to become loose over time—especially in young, active patients who generally put more strain on the joints. A better alternative appears to be cementless joints. These porous implants allow the bone to grow into the artificial joint, making for a firmer fit.

Total hip and knee replacements have a very high success rate. Artificial shoulders and elbows are done less frequently. Other procedures include total wrist and ankle joint replacements and also artificial finger joint implants.

You can improve your chances for success by choosing your doctor and hospital carefully. Be sure to ask your doctor how many times he or she has performed your particular procedure. The more familiar your doctor is with the operation, the better the chance of a good outcome.

Since artificial joints inevitably wear out, it's sometimes advisable to put off the procedure as long as possible—especially in younger patients, who might require several replacements of the same joint over the course of a lifetime. Such patients can forestall a joint replacement by instead undergoing another surgical procedure called an osteotomy, which involves cutting a bone adjacent to a joint. By changing the angle at which bones in the joint meet, an osteotomy can redistribute stresses on the affected joint (typically a hip or knee), so that the joint can continue to function for a longer time.

Chapter 4

The One-Two Supplement Punch

An extensive amount of research—some fifteen clinical studies—has shown that two dietary supplements, glucosamine and chondroitin sulfate, can offer you what you've been searching for: not just relief from the pain and other vexing symptoms of osteoarthritis without recourse to toxic drugs, but also a way to halt the disease in its tracks and even rebuild lost cartilage.

In fact, these supplements offer so much promise for treating and even reversing osteoarthritis that *The Arthritis Solution* has made them the focus of its three-prong strategy against osteoarthritis. You may never have heard of them until you picked up this book. That's not surprising, since glucosamine and chondroitin sulfate have not received the attention they deserve, for several reasons.

First of all, the studies of glucosamine and chondroitin sulfate have almost all been carried out in other countries, chiefly Germany, Italy, and France. American medicine often discounts the significance of research in other countries, and the research on these supplements is no exception. Until just recently, U.S.

researchers largely ignored what their overseas colleagues have had to say about these supplements, perhaps in part because some of the work appeared in foreign-language medical journals.

Fortunately, the word has finally gotten out, and indifference has changed to enthusiasm. As of this writing, two controlled clinical trials are now underway in this country, testing a combination of glucosamine and chondroitin sulfate on people with osteoarthritis. Some results should be available by the end of 1997.

The second reason that glucosamine and chondroitin sulfate are relatively unknown is that they're "only" dietary supplements and are not classified as drugs—which may actually be for the best. Each year, Americans spend billions of dollars on steroids and NSAIDs for the treatment of osteoarthritis pain, yet these drugs do nothing to remedy the cartilage damage that's at the heart of osteoarthritis. In fact, the drugs mainly used to treat osteoarthritis—aspirin and other NSAIDs—can cause gastrointestinal bleeding that leads to thousands of deaths each year, particularly among arthritis sufferers who must take them regularly and in high doses for relief.

By contrast, glucosamine and chondroitin sulfate are produced in small amounts by our own bodies, they're present in some of the foods we eat, and they have no significant side effects. In short, these are safe, natural substances. But as "mere" dietary supplements, glucosamine and chondroitin sulfate don't get the respect—from doctors or pharmaceutical companies—that they might otherwise receive if they were drugs.

Much of the research on new treatments is funded by pharmaceutical companies, which stand to profit handsomely by creating a drug in the laboratory, patenting it, and carrying out the costly research and development necessary to bring it to market—costs estimated at between $300 million and $500 million for a new drug that ultimately gains approval. But natural substances such as glucosamine and chondroitin sulfate can't be patented. So it's understandable that pharmaceutical companies have shown little interest in funding research that by now could have made these supplements mainstream treatments for osteoarthritis.

This lack of interest by the drug companies toward dietary supplements is matched by the disinterest shown by doctors. Only in the past couple of years have more than a handful of medical schools offered courses in nutrition to the doctors they train. So the idea of nutritional therapy in the form of supplements is foreign to most physicians. When patients ask their doctors about the merits of taking a dietary supplement, the most enthusiastic response they're likely to get is, "Well, at least it probably won't hurt you."

Finally, the U.S. Food and Drug Administration's stance toward supplements hasn't done much to increase the public's appreciation for these substances. Historically, the FDA has taken a dim view of supplements, sometimes cracking down hard on manufacturers that dared to make therapeutic claims for them.

These regulatory actions have sometimes served the public interest—particularly when claims have been obviously bogus (that blue-green algae can cure cancer, for example) or when the supplement posed a health hazard (megadoses of vitamin A marketed to pregnant women). But there has also been a downside to the FDA's hostility toward supplements: It has interfered with the public's awareness of truly worthwhile dietary supplements such as glucosamine and chondroitin sulfate. Despite the proven therapeutic benefits of these supplements, manufacturers have been restricted in terms of the therapeutic claims they've been able to make for them.

By informing people like you how these products can help relieve their osteoarthritis, this book may help to rescue glucosamine and chondroitin sulfate from their undeserved obscurity. If you're like most people with osteoarthritis, the news about glucosamine and chondroitin sulfate may well be the first good news you've ever gotten about your condition.

A New Era in Osteoarthritis Treatment

Your osteoarthritis may cause a slight twinge in your knee. Your neighbor, on the other hand, may have osteoarthritis of the hip so crippling that she needs a joint replacement operation. But while people differ widely regarding the seriousness of their osteoarthritis, you can bet they've all heard some discouraging words when they've sought treatment: "We can help you manage the pain," their doctors have told them, "but beyond that there's not much we can do for you." No wonder so many people become depressed after being told they have osteoarthritis. They figure they have little to look forward to but years of increasing pain and disability.

By the time someone with osteoarthritis notices pain and stiffness and makes an appointment with a doctor, the disease is typically at an advanced stage and joints are severely damaged. So it's not surprising that researchers have long regarded osteoarthritis as a relentlessly degenerative disease, in which cartilage simply erodes steadily over the years until bone grinds against bone.

Fortunately, medicine's understanding of osteoarthritis has changed drastically over the past few years. The disease is not regarded as the inevitable, passive process it was long thought to be.

Instead, studies have shown that the joints *can* repair themselves by producing new cartilage to replace that which has been lost or damaged. A treatment that can enhance cartilage's ability to repair itself could slow down or even reverse the disease. The aim now is to intervene in osteoarthritis at an early stage, in time to keep joints from becoming severely damaged. And the best candidates for accomplishing that task are glucosamine sulfate and chondroitin sulfate, the nutritional supplements that are the focus of this book.

Glucosamine and chondroitin sulfate don't just put a Band-Aid on the pain and other symptoms of osteoarthritis the way the NSAIDs and other drugs do. Instead, they actually get inside cartilage—preserving what's left of it, repairing damaged areas, and preventing its further breakdown. In short, these supplements are light years better than any drugs you've been taking. They affect the disease process itself, by putting an end to cartilage destruction and actually pitching in to rebuild it.

Why They Work

The new understanding of osteoarthritis has come from a new appreciation of cartilage, the site in the body where osteoarthritis occurs. Once regarded as simple and inert, cartilage turns out to be a dynamic tissue seething with metabolic activity, with cartilage synthesis and destruction occurring simultaneously.

Healthy cartilage is a stable tissue because the rate

at which the body makes it is equal to the rate at which it's broken down. But in osteoarthritis the balance shifts: While cartilage-destroying enzymes are proceeding full speed ahead, the body doesn't produce cartilage fast enough to keep up—a slowdown that may be due to aging. If this one-sided battle continues, cartilage will eventually erode away. But fortunately, this is the point where the one-two punch of glucosamine sulfate and chondroitin sulfate can make a big difference.

Working in combination, glucosamine and chondroitin sulfate speed up the manufacture of new cartilage while at the same time suppressing cartilage destruction. It amounts to nothing less than intervening to halt a disease and helping the body to heal itself. For you to really appreciate what these supplements can do for you, we need to take a look inside the cartilage, where osteoarthritis occurs and where these two supplements work to stop it.

A Tangled Web

Think of cartilage as a spiderweb—not some thin, two-dimensional web but a massive web of the kind that fills a broom closet that you haven't opened for years. Scattered throughout this huge web are the relatively small number of "spiders" responsible for creating and maintaining it. These are the cartilage cells, also known as chondrocytes. This cartilage "web" consists of two types of "silk"—the two basic components that are spun out by the spiderlike cartilage cells and that provide cartilage with its structure, shape, and strength. These two key components of cartilage are collagen and proteoglycan molecules.

You've probably heard of collagen. Tough and fibrous, it's the most common protein in the body and also the body's structural "glue," helping to hold the cells and tissues of the body together. Collagen's rod-shaped fibers form an important part of the skin, tendons, and bones. And as a key part of cartilage, collagen provides cartilage with its strength and its ability to resist being pulled apart by pressure and other forces.

Proteoglycans, the partner of collagen in forming cartilage's weblike structure, provide cartilage with the flexibility it needs to make it a good shock absorber. The proteoglycans accomplish this through their extraordinary ability to attract many times their weight in water. In fact, just as a spiderweb is mostly air, up to eighty percent of human cartilage *is* water, which comes from the synovial fluid that bathes the joints.

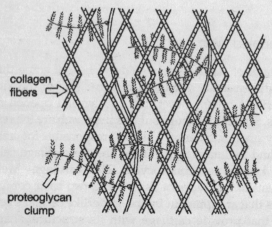

collagen fibers ⇨

⇧ proteoglycan clump

Cartilage

A proteoglycan molecule is referred to as a macro-molecule because of its huge size. Each one resembles a furry caterpillar, with hundreds of molecules (known as side chains) jutting out like fur from the proteoglycan's protein "backbone."

In healthy cartilage, up to fifty of the caterpillarlike proteoglycan molecules fasten onto a long molecule called hyaluronic acid to form a "megacaterpillar" clump of proteoglycans. Most of the proteoglycans in cartilage are found in this form. Each proteoglycan clump has numerous side chains provided by its individual proteoglycan molecules; with their negative electrical charges, these side chains repel each other while also acting as magnets for pulling water molecules into cartilage. Proteoglycans pull in the right amount of water to give cartilage the consistency of a stiff gel, able to take a pounding without suffering damage.

If cartilage is the battlefield in osteoarthritis, then the proteoglycans are Ground Zero—where the destruction of cartilage is truly centered. In osteoarthritis the proteoglycans in cartilage appear to dwindle away, due primarily to destructive enzymes produced by the cartilage cells. As the proteoglycans disappear, so too does their knack for binding the proper amount of water within cartilage to keep it supple. Instead, cartilage becomes waterlogged, soft, and fragile and ultimately wears away.

Glucosamine and chondroitin sulfate help to defeat osteoarthritis by supporting the all-important proteoglycans. Glucosamine acts offensively to bolster the supply of proteoglycans and to repair and rebuild cartilage that has been damaged or lost. Chondroitin, on the other hand, is chiefly a defensive player that works to suppress the enzymes that eat away at cartilage.

The Glory of Glucosamine

Picture that caterpillarlike proteoglycan molecule, bristling with its hundreds of furlike side chains that pull water into cartilage. The key raw material for making these crucial side chains is glucosamine, which the body obtains in one of two ways: It can synthesize its own, or it can use the glucosamine that it obtains from food (particularly meat with gristle) or from supplements.

When you swallow it, glucosamine is very efficiently absorbed. In fact, about ninety percent of the amount that you swallow ends up in your bloodstream. But does it go where it can do the most good? Researchers have actually addressed that question. They put a radioactive "tag" on glucosamine molecules and then fed the glucosamine to animals so the molecules could be traced after the animals swallowed them. When they looked for the tagged molecules of glucosamine, the researchers found that they had selectively been taken up by the cartilage at the ends of the animals' bones—just where they were supposed to go.

Once swallowed, the glucosamine does more than become incorporated into new side chains for the proteoglycans. Its mere presence stimulates the chondrocytes (cartilage cells) to spring into action and start churning out more of these proteoglycans; the more glucosamine sulfate available, the more proteoglycans the cartilage cells will produce. Finally, glucosamine also appears to stimulate cartilage cells to produce more collagen, the other major component of cartilage. In these ways, glucosamine sulfate helps to rebuild the cartilage that's been lost due to osteoarthritis.

Putting Glucosamine to the Test

Now that you've read how glucosamine comes to the rescue of eroding cartilage, you're probably saying to yourself, "This all sounds good on paper, but does it translate into relieving my morning stiffness and pain?" The answer is a resounding *yes*. And to prove it, there are ten clinical studies in which glucosamine was tested on actual osteoarthritis patients. Most of the studies were very well designed, so their conclusions can be accepted as being scientifically valid. Thanks to these studies, glucosamine has now become a standard treatment for osteoarthritis in Europe.

Nearly all of the glucosamine studies were "placebo controlled," meaning that some patients were treated with glucosamine sulfate while others received an inert, dummy medicine. By comparing the results from the treatment with those observed in the control group, researchers can be sure that benefits observed are truly due to the therapy and not just to the "placebo effect"—the proven ability of sugar pills to make people feel better simply because they think they're receiving a drug. In addition, most studies were "double blind," meaning that, during the study, neither the researchers nor the patients knew who was in the control group and who was in the treatment group.

These clinical studies have shown that glucosamine offers osteoarthritis patients the following major benefits:

Significant Pain Relief. If any one message comes through loud and clear from these studies, it's that glucosamine can relieve the pain your osteoarthritis is causing you. A prime example is a study done in Milan, Italy, involving eighty patients, all of whom had suffered from severe osteoarthritis for a long time. In this thirty-day double-blind study, patients were given either 1.5 grams of glucosamine daily or a placebo. The researchers measured the patients' pain, joint tenderness, swelling, and the range of motion of their joints each week. The results were clear-cut:

- Seventy-two percent of the patients treated with glucosamine experienced measurable improvement in symptoms versus only thirty-six percent of the patients taking the placebo—a significant difference.
- The patients taking the glucosamine needed only twenty days for the severity of their symptoms to be reduced by half. By contrast, those patients on the placebo needed an average of thirty days for the same improvement.
- By the end of the study, one out of five patients taking glucosamine was totally symptom-free, *compared with none of the forty patients taking the placebo.*
- When asked to assess the results, the doctors participating in the study (who didn't know which patients were on glucosamine and which were on the placebo) graded twenty-nine of the forty patients receiving glucosamine as attaining "excellent" or "good" results, compared with only seventeen of the forty who were in the placebo group.

The researchers credited glucosamine's ability to rebuild damaged cartilage for the striking improvement in symptoms that was noted in the study.

Fast Relief of Symptoms. Another double-blind study, this one done in the Philippines, involved twenty patients with osteoarthritis of the knee. Ten of the patients were given 1500 milligrams of glucosamine daily while the other ten received a placebo. After eight weeks, the differences were clear: significant improvements in pain, joint tenderness, and swelling in the patients receiving glucosamine compared with the patients on the placebo. But most impressive of all, the average glucosamine-treated patients showed clinical improvement after only fourteen days of treatment, but it took the average patient on the placebo forty days to show clinical improvement.

Excellent Safety. In another double-blind Italian study, glucosamine once again far outshone a placebo medication in providing pain relief and relieving joint stiffness. But of particular interest, the glucosamine was administered in a potent form—intravenously—to patients who were seriously ill with circulatory disorders, liver ailments, diabetes, and lung disease. But despite their ill health, none of the patients experienced adverse effects from the glucosamine.

When taken orally—the way most people take it—glucosamine has also proven quite safe. In all the clinical studies, people who took glucosamine supplements had no more problems of any kind, including heartburn or other gastrointestinal problems, than did their counterparts who were taking placebos.

Produces Long-lasting Effects. In a large Portuguese study, more than 1200 patients with osteoarthritis were given 1500 milligrams of glucosamine daily for an average of fifty days. As in other studies, there was overall relief in pain and other symptoms—in this case by an average of seventy percent. But equally impressive was how long the relief from symptoms persisted: Patients continued to experience relief from six to twelve weeks after treatment with glucosamine had stopped.

Works as Well as Drugs. In another Portuguese study, glucosamine was compared with ibuprofen, the NSAID marketed in prescription form as Motrin and available over the counter as Advil and Nuprin. In this double-blind study, patients with osteoarthritis of the knee were treated for eight weeks with either 1500 milligrams of glucosamine daily or with 1500 milligrams of ibuprofen (slightly above the 1200 milligrams recommended for over-the-counter ibuprofen).

For both groups, pain levels dropped significantly over the first two weeks—and, in fact, pain relief was more rapid in the ibuprofen group. But after the two-week mark, ibuprofen seemed to lose some effectiveness and was soon overtaken by glucosamine. By the end of the eight-week study, patients treated with glucosamine reported significantly better pain relief than those on ibuprofen. In addition, knee swelling subsided in twenty percent of patients treated with glucosamine compared with none of the people on ibuprofen. Overall, twenty-nine percent more patients in the glucosamine group had good outcomes than in the ibuprofen group.

Another study comparing glucosamine and ibuprofen, carried out by researchers in Germany and Italy, served to underline glucosamine's safety. This double-blind study, published in 1994, involved two hundred patients hospitalized with osteoarthritis of the knee. Every day over a four-week period, patients received either 1500 milligrams of glucosamine or 1200 milligrams of ibuprofen.

As in the previous study, both groups experienced pain relief; but for the first two weeks, relief was more pronounced among people taking ibuprofen. After that, however, the people taking glucosamine "caught up," and, in the study's final two weeks, glucosamine proved to be as effective as ibuprofen in relieving symptoms. Glucosamine was much better tolerated by the patients: Out of one hundred patients taking ibuprofen, thirty-five complained of side effects throughout treatment and seven of them dropped out of the study; but in the glucosamine group, only six patients reported any problems and only one person dropped out.

Rebuilds Cartilage. Glucosamine's ability to rebuild cartilage is more than theoretical conjecture: There is microscropic evidence that it actually happens. In the Milan study described above, in which patients with severe osteoarthritis took 1.5 grams of glucosamine orally for thirty days, samples of cartilage from patients in the two groups were compared under an electron microscope. Samples from the glucosamine-treated patients appeared to be healthy cartilage, while samples from patients in the placebo group exhibited the erosion that is typical in osteoarthritis.

Chondroitin Sulfate to the Rescue

The second important supplement that has proven beneficial to osteoarthritis sufferers, chondroitin sulfate, occurs naturally in cartilage. In fact, molecules of chondroitin sulfate make up most of the proteoglycan "side chains" we mentioned earlier—the ones that act like magnets for pulling water into cartilage.

When researchers began studying chondroitin sulfate supplements, they hoped that chondroitin molecules, when swallowed, would act as "replacement parts" for the chondroitin sulfate side chains that are lost due to osteoarthritis. But since chondroitin sulfate molecules are huge—far bigger than glucosamine sulfate—the question "Does it really get absorbed when you swallow it?" was front and center on their research agenda.

Several studies, involving both human volunteers and experimental animals, have shown that about seventy percent of the chondroitin does get absorbed from the intestine into the blood. Furthermore, some of that chondroitin reaches the synovial fluid of the joint and becomes incorporated into cartilage.

While chondroitin sulfate taken as a supplement does help to rebuild cartilage, it also does something else that may be even more important: It blocks the destructive enzymes in cartilage that break down the all-important proteoglycan molecules. That should help to reduce any inflammation that may be present inside the joint. But more crucially, by curbing cartilage breakdown, chondroitin sulfate also helps to slow down the process of osteoarthritis and even helps to rebuild cartilage.

Chondroitin sulfate has been the focus of several clinical trials, and the results indicate that this supplement lives up to its billing as a cartilage protector and enhancer. The studies have found that chondroitin sulfate offers the following benefits:

Safety and Effectiveness. To qualify for a 1991 study in Naples, Italy, patients had to have at least five of these signs or symptoms: evidence of osteoarthritis on an X ray; a typical clinical history of osteoarthritis; swelling of at least one joint; reddening of at least one joint; extreme sensitivity to pressure on at least one joint; pain when resting or moving at least one joint; and no sign of any other type of arthritis. In this six-month study, two hundred patients received either 1200 milligrams of oral chondroitin sulfate daily or a daily injection of 100 milligrams of chondroitin sulfate. At the study's end, researchers concluded that "the results showed a considerable improvement both in pain and mobility. No relevant side effects were found."

Long-term Relief. A French study published in 1992 assessed chondroitin sulfate's pain-relieving ability. In this double-blind study, 120 patients with osteoarthritis of the knees and hips received either oral chondroitin sulfate or a placebo for three months. The researcher assessed the patients' conditions by tracking their need for NSAID pain relievers. At the end of the three months, consumption of NSAIDs had decreased significantly in the chondroitin group compared with the placebo group—indicating that people taking chondroitin experienced much better pain relief. Equally notable was the sustained relief afforded the patients taking the chondroitin: They were still experiencing relief when they were reevaluated two months after the study had ended.

Improved Joint Movement. Another double-blind French study involved 129 osteoarthritis patients who were treated daily for six months either with oral chondroitin sulfate or a placebo. "Highly significant differences in favor of chondroitin sulfate" were noted after the first month and persisted throughout the six-month study. In particular, the patients taking the chondroitin had significantly better joint movement than the people in the placebo group.

Catch the Synergy

So you have two useful supplements against osteo-arthritis. One of them, glucosamine, works offensively by rebuilding cartilage. The other, chondroitin sulfate, helps against osteoarthritis mainly in a defensive way, by inhibiting enzymes that break down cartilage. Why not combine both supplements in the same capsule?

Nutramax Laboratories of Baltimore came up with that idea and in 1992 began marketing a combination supplement called Cosamin. Now the company also offers a double-strength variant called Cosamin DS. Each capsule of Cosamin DS contains 500 milligrams of glucosamine hydrochloride and 400 milligrams of chondroitin sulfate. As shown in the table on page 76, several other companies are now marketing combination products containing these two supplements.

Judging by what each ingredient offers on its own, researchers are hopeful that the combination will have a synergistic effect in cartilage—meaning that the impact of the supplements acting together will far exceed the additive benefits from giving each one individually.

So far, the combination of glucosamine and chondroitin has been tested only in dogs, horses, and other animals that share with humans the tendency to develop osteoarthritis. The results of these studies show that the combination product is promising and quite safe to use.

Studies testing the combination in humans are now underway. One of them, being carried out in North Carolina, is a double-blind, placebo-controlled study involving one hundred patients with osteoarthritis of the knee who are receiving either the combination product or a placebo. Another study, also placebo-controlled, is being carried out by U.S. Department of Defense researchers and involves forty elite Navy commandos known as SEALS who have osteoarthritis of the knee or the back.

Should you buy glucosamine, chondroitin, or a combination of the two? The studies published to date indicate that you're likely to see benefits whichever option you choose. Either singly or in combination, these supplements are not only effective in relieving the symptoms of osteoarthritis but are also quite safe. But since they do work in different ways to rebuild cartilage, taking both might be the best choice. You could take either a two-in-one combination product or buy bottles of both glucosamine and chondroitin sulfate supplements.

If you decide to take the supplements, you'll have a dizzying array of products to choose from. The table provided here should help to sort things out for you. It lists many of the glucosamine, chondroitin, and combination products now being sold, their suggested retail prices, and other information, including how you can order these products by mail.

You don't need a prescription for any of these products, although some brands are sold only to health care professionals, who then dispense them to their patients. Before you embark on a regimen of these supplements, it's a good idea to consult your doctor to make sure that they're appropriate for your particular arthritic problem and your general medical condition.

In the next chapter, we tell you what you need to know when you're starting out on these dietary supplements: recommended doses, how to fit the supplements into your overall strategy against osteoarthritis, and when you can expect to notice improvements in your symptoms.

COMBINATION GLUCOSAMINE/CHONDROITIN PRODUCTS

Product Name	Manufacturer	Form	Amount per Capsule/Tablet (mg)	Capsules/Tablets Recommended Daily	No. of Capsules/Tablets per Bottle	Suggested Retail Price	Comments
Chondroitin Sulfate/ Glucosamine Sulfate	Optimal Nutrients, Foster City, CA 800-966-8874	Capsule	400 mg chondroitin sulfate and 500 mg glucosamine sulfate	Three	60 and 90	$30.95 and $45.49	Sold in health food stores and by mail order
Cosamin DS	Nutramax Laboratories, Baltimore, MD 800-925-5187	Capsule	500 mg glucosamine HCl and 400 mg chondroitin sulfate	Three to Four	90 and 180	$60 and $100	Sold only through health care professionals and in pharmacies. Lower-strength formulation (Cosamin) also available. Call Nutramax for a list of pharmacies that provide Cosamin DS by mail order. Shop around, since retail prices vary considerably

GluChon 900	Thompson Nutritional Products, Boca Raton, FL 800-421-1192	Tablet	500 mg glucosamine HCl and 400 mg chondroitin sulfate	Three to Four	60	$38.95	Available in health food stores or by mail order from these distributors: L&H Vitamins, 800-221-1152, East Coast; Linberg Nutrition, 800-338-7979, West Coast; or Swanson Health Products, 800-437-4148, Midwest
Glucosamine Chondroitin Complex	Solgar Vitamin and Herb Co., Leonia, NJ 201-944-2311	Tablet	500 mg glucosamine sulfate and 500 mg chondroitin sulfate	Two	60	$30.32	Sold in health food stores or by mail order from Wilner Chemists 800-633-1106
Glucosamine Complex	Country Life, Hauppauge, NY 800-851-2200, 800-645-5768 (East Coast)	Capsule	125 mg glucosamine sulfate, 125 mg n-acetyl glucosamine, 125 mg glucosamine HCl, and 125 mg chondroitin sulfate	Two to Four	50 and 100	$20.05 and $35	Sold in health food stores and by mail order from The Vitamin Shoppe 800-223-1216

COMBINATION GLUCOSAMINE/CHONDROITIN PRODUCTS (cont.)

Product Name	Manufacturer	Form	Amount per Capsule/ Tablet (mg)	Capsules/ Tablets Recom- mended Daily	No. of Capsules/ Tablets per Bottle	Suggested Retail Price	Comments
Joint Fuel	TwinLab, Ronkonkoma, NY 800-645-5626 (516-467-3140 in NY)		250 mg glucosamine sulfate and 17 mg chondroitin sulfate	Six	60	$26.50	Sold in most health food stores and available by mail order from L&H Vitamins 800-221-1152
Natural Pain Relief Formula	Inholtra Natural Ltd., Kennebunk, ME 800-808-7266	Capsule	167 mg n-acetyl glucosamine, 167 mg glucosamine sulfate, and 67 mg chondroitin sulfate	Three to Nine	90	$46.95	Sold in health food stores and by mail order
Nutritional Support for Joints	The Vitamin Shoppe, North Bergen, NJ 800-223-1216	Tablets	250 mg glucosamine sulfate and 17 mg chondroitin sulfate	Six	100 and 300	$19.95 and $49.95	Sold in Vitamin Shoppe stores and by mail order

Perfect Joint Combination	Healthy Origins, Pittsburgh, PA	Capsule	250 mg D-glucosamine sulfate and 200 mg chondroitin sulfate	Four to Eight	60	$38.95	Sold in GNC stores
Nutri-Joint	Vitamin Research Products, Carson City, NV 800-877-2447	Capsule	300 mg glucosamine HCl, 100 mg n-acetyl glucosamine, and 300 mg chondroitin sulfate	Three	90	$38.95	Available mostly in West Coast health food stores and by mail order
Osteo-Bi-Flex 450	Sundown Vitamins, Boca Raton, FL 800-327-0908	Tablet	250 mg glucosamine HCl and 200 mg chondroitin sulfate	Six for first 60 days, then three to six	48	$15.99	Sold in pharmacies and food and retail chain stores. Contains the same formula used in Cosamin DS but in a lower dosage form
Rehab Support	Professional Botanicals, Ogden, UT 801-479-6533	Capsule	500 mg glucosamine chlorohydrate and 50 mg chondroitin sulfate	Three	60	$24	Sold only through health care professionals

GLUCOSAMINE PRODUCTS

Product Name	Manufacturer	Form	Amount per Capsule/ Tablet (mg)	Capsules/ Tablets Recom- mended Daily	No. of Capsules/ Tablets per Bottle	Suggested Retail Price	Comments
Advanced Glucosamine Complex	Solgar Vitamin and Herb Co., Leonia, NJ 201-944-2311	Tablet	200 mg glucosamine HCl, 200 mg glucosamine sulfate, and 200 mg n-acetyl glucosamine	One or Two	30 and 60	$8.95 and $16.56	Sold in health food stores and by mail order from Wilner Chemists 800-633-1106
Arth-X Plus	Trace Minerals Research, Roy, UT 800-624-7145	Tablet	87 mg glucosamine sulfate	Two to Six	90, 180, 360	$21.39, $41.50, $78.90	Sold in most health food stores and from 11 mail order suppliers. Call company for name of store in your area that carries Arth-X Plus or the name of a mail order supplier
Enhanced Glucosamine Sulfate	General Nutrition Corp., Pittsburgh, PA 412-288-4600	Capsule	375 mg D-glucosamine sulfate	Four	60	$19.99	Products sold only in GNC stores

Flexi-Factors	Country Life, Hauppauge, NY 800-851-2200, 800-645-5768 (East Coast)	Tablet	63 mg n-acetyl glucosamine and 63 mg glucosamine sulfate	Three	50	$16.50	Sold in most health food stores and by mail order
Glucosamine Complex	Vitamin Research Products, Carson City, NV 800-877-2447	Capsule	250 mg glucosamine HCl, 250 mg n-acetyl glucosamine	Three	90	$28.95	Sold mostly in West Coast health food stores and by mail order
Glucosamine HCL with N-A-G	KAL, Park City, UT 801-655-6003	Capsule	500 mg glucosamine HCl and 150 mg n-acetyl glucosamine	Two to Four	120	$35.04	Sold in health food stores
Glucosamine Mega 1000	Jarrow Formulas, Los Angeles, CA 800-726-0886	Tablet	1,000 mg glucosamine HCl	One or Two	100	$22.49	Products sold in health food stores (mainly on West Coast) and by mail order from Vitamin Trader 800-334-9310 or Omega Nutrition 800-661-3529

GLUCOSAMINE PRODUCTS (cont.)

Product Name	Manufacturer	Form	Amount per Capsule/ Tablet (mg)	Capsules/ Tablets Recommended Daily	No. of Capsules/ Tablets per Bottle	Suggested Retail Price	Comments
Glucosamine Sulfate	Solgar Vitamin and Herb Co., Leonia, NJ 201-944-2311	Tablet	1000 mg glucosamine sulfate	One or Two	30 and 60	$18.32 and $34.80	Sold in health food stores and by mail order from Wilner Chemists 800-633-1106
Glucosamine Sulfate	TwinLab, Ronkonkoma, NY 800-645-5626 (516-467-3140 in NY)	Capsule	750 mg glucosamine sulfate	Two	30, 60, 90	$14.80, $27.96, $40.76	Sold in most health food stores and by mail order from L&H Vitamins 800-221-1152
Glucosamine Sulfate	Nutricology, San Leandro, CA 800-545-9960	Capsule	500 mg glucosamine sulfate	One to Four	90	$29.00	Sold in health food stores and by mail order
Glucosamine Sulfate	Great Earth, Ontario, CA 800-284-8243	Tablet	500 mg glucosamine sulfate	One to Three	60	$14.39	Sold in Great Earth stores or by mail order
Glucosamine Sulfate	Tyler Encapsulations, Gresham, OR 800-869-9705	Capsule	500 mg glucosamine sulfate	Three	60 and 120	$20 and $38	Product is sold only to health care professionals

Glucosamine Sulfate 500	Jarrow Formulas, Los Angeles, CA 800-726-0886	Capsule	500 mg glucosamine sulfate	One to Four	100	$27.95	Products sold in health food stores (mainly on West Coast) and by mail order from Vitamin Trader 800-334-9310 or Omega Nutrition 800-661-3529
Glucosamine sulfate 500	The Vitamin Shoppe, North Bergen, NJ 800-223-1216	Capsule	500 mg glucosamine sulfate	Three	60 and 120	$15.95 and $26.95	Sold in Vitamin Shoppe stores and by mail order
GS-500	Enzymatic Therapy, Green Bay, WI 800-783-2286	Capsule	500 mg glucosamine sulfate	Three	120	$40.00	Sold in health food stores
Joint Care	Jarrow Formulas, Los Angeles, CA 800-726-0886	Tablet	1,500 mg glucosamine HCl	Two to Four	120	$29.95	Products sold in health food stores (mainly on West Coast) and by mail order from Vitamin Trader 800-334-9310 or Omega Nutrition 800-661-3529
Joint Factors	TwinLab, Ronkonkoma, NY 800-645-5626 (516-467-3140 in NY)	Capsule	375 mg glucosamine sulfate	Four	60	$19.97	Sold in most health food stores and by mail order from L&H Vitamins 800-221-1152

GLUCOSAMINE PRODUCTS (cont.)

Product Name	Manufacturer	Form	Amount per Capsule/ Tablet (mg)	Capsules/ Tablets Recom- mended Daily	No. of Capsules/ Tablets per Bottle	Suggested Retail Price	Comments
Opti-GS 750	Optimal Nutrients, Foster City, CA 800-966-8874	Capsule	750 mg glucosamine sulfate	Two to Four	60, 120, 180	$22.95, $42.95, $62.95	Sold in health food stores; also available in dosage forms of 500 mg per capsule and 1,000 mg per capsule
Mobil-Ease	Prevail, Gresham, OR 800-248-0885	Capsule	500 mg glucosamine sulfate	Two to Three	60	$22.95	Sold in health food stores and by mail order
N-acetyl glucosamine	Jarrow Formulas, Los Angeles, CA 800-726-0886	Capsule	750 mg n-acetyl glucosamine	One to Three	60 and 120	$23.95 and $38.95	Products sold in health food stores (mainly on West Coast) and by mail order from Vitamin Trader 800-334-9310 or Omega Nutrition 800-661-3529
Ultra Glucosamine Sulfate	The Vitamin Shoppe, North Bergen, NJ 800-223-1216	Capsule	1000 mg glucosamine sulfate	Three	60 and 120	$23.95 and $42.95	Sold in Vitamin Shoppe stores and by mail order
Ultra Glucosamine 600	Nature's Plus, Melville, NY 800-645-9500	Tablet	600 mg glucosamine sulfate	Three	60	$25.25	Sold in health food stores; call 800-937-0500 for a store in your area that carries it
Glucosamine HCl	Nature's Way, Springville, UT 800-9-NATURE	Capsule	500 mg glucosamine HCl	Three	90	$17.49	Sold in most health food stores and by mail order

CHONDROITIN SULFATE PRODUCTS

Product Name	Manufacturer	Form	Amount per Capsule/Tablet (mg)	Capsules/Tablets Recommended Daily	No. of Capsules/Tablets per Bottle	Suggested Retail Price	Comments
Bovine Trachea Cartilage/ chondroitin sulfate	Jarrow Formulas, Los Angeles, CA 800-726-0886	Capsule	222 mg chondroitin sulfate	Seven to Twelve	120	$22.95	Products sold in health food stores (mainly on West Coast) and by mail order from Vitamin Trader 800-334-9310 or Omega Nutrition 800-661-3529
Chondroitin-4-sulphate	Ecological Formulas, Concord, CA 800-888-4585	Capsule	250 mg	Two	60	$15.95	Sold in some health food stores and pharmacies and by mail order
Chondroitin Sulfate	American Biologics, Chula Vista, CA 800-227-4473	Capsule	300 mg chondroitin sulfate	One to Three	60	$26.90	Also available in 500 mg capsules. Sold in some health food stores and by mail order
Chondroitin Sulfate	Natrol, Chatsworth, CA 800-326-1520	Capsule	500 mg chondroitin sulfate	One to Two	60	$39.98	Sold in health food stores and by mail order from L&H Vitamins 800-221-1152

CHONDROITIN SULFATE PRODUCTS (cont.)

Product Name	Manufacturer	Form	Amount per Capsule/ Tablet (mg)	Capsules/ Tablets Recom- mended Daily	No. of Capsules/ Tablets per Bottle	Suggested Retail Price	Comments
Chondroitin Sulfate-A	The Vitamin Shoppe, North Bergen, NJ 800-223-1216	Tablet	500 mg chondroitin sulfate	Two or more	100	$39.95	Sold in Vitamin Shoppe stores and by mail order
CSA	TwinLab, Ronkonkoma, NY 800-645-5626 (516-467-3140 in NY)	Capsule	250 mg chondroitin sulfate	One	60	$23.95	Sold in most health food stores
Bovine Cartilage Extract	Vitamin Research Products, Carson City, NV 800-877-2447	Capsule	500 mg chondroitin sulfate	Two to Ten	90	$27.95	Available mostly in West Coast health food stores and by mail order

Chapter 5

Devising Your Supplement Strategy

If you've read the preceding chapter, you'll know that you now have a tremendous opportunity to do something about your osteoarthritis. By using a clinically proven pair of dietary supplements, you can ease your symptoms and synthesize new cartilage to replace cartilage that has been lost—and you can accomplish both of these goals safely and naturally, without the harmful side effects often associated with drugs.

Now that you know what glucosamine and chondroitin sulfate can do for you, it's time to take action. From the clinical work that has been done so far, it appears that your best tactic for overcoming osteoarthritis is to use the two dietary supplements in combination, although as we'll see there may be reasons for using them singly.

To be successful in achieving any goal, whether it be learning to play tennis or overcoming osteoarthritis, being motivated is absolutely essential. By reading this book and learning about glucosamine and chondroitin sulfate, you've shown that you've got what it takes in that department. But to actually realize your objectives of less osteoarthritis pain and better mobility through the use of these dietary supplements, you'll also need another quality, and that's patience. What is truly worthwhile is rarely achieved overnight, and you must keep that in mind when you begin using these two supplements. You've got to be patient while they make your joints better places for your bones to move around in.

Although you may only recently have experienced pain and stiffness in your joints, the degradation of cartilage has probably been going on for years, only now having progressed to the point where you're feeling the symptoms of bone rubbing against bone. So it may take some time for glucosamine and chondroitin sulfate to turn this situation around.

The pain relief drugs, such as the NSAIDs commonly prescribed for osteoarthritis, can certainly work faster than chondroitin or glucosamine sulfate—the clinical trials comparing the supplements with NSAIDs have shown that. But these drugs can only relieve the *symptoms* of osteoarthritis; they do nothing about the underlying disease process—the insidious destruction of cartilage—that is causing those symptoms. As a matter of fact, there is some evidence that long-term use of certain NSAIDs can damage cartilage.

By contrast, chondroitin sulfate and glucosamine take longer to produce noticeable benefits because these dietary supplements work in a much more basic—and constructive—way. They help to halt and even reverse disease progression by actually rebuilding the cartilage that has worn away over the years. And it's this restoration of the protective, cushioning cartilage that yields the pain relief and increased range of motion that so many people who use glucosamine and chondroitin sulfate are now experiencing.

You Can't Hurry Cartilage

How long before you're likely to notice the benefits that these supplements offer? The answer will vary, determined in part by you and your physiology in general and, in particular, the cartilage at the ends of your bones, where these supplements will begin their restoration process.

Think of the new cartilage you'll be building as delicate buds emerging after a long winter has worn away much of the protective covering in the surrounding landscape. How soon those buds of cartilage take hold, flourish, and ultimately become a luxuriant covering for your bones depends on a number of factors, including:

How Much Cartilage Needs to Be Replaced. Cartilage wears away over many years, so it's too much to expect that it can be rebuilt overnight. Generally, the people who do best with these supplements are those who have mild to moderate rather than severe cases of osteoarthritis. The more cartilage you've already lost, the longer it will take before you start to notice some improvement in your symptoms of osteoarthritis.

How Old You Are. As we get older, all our bodily repair processes start to slow down. Just as it takes more time to recover from surgery, it also takes longer for cartilage repair to occur. On top of that, older people are likely to have more of a cartilage "deficit" than younger people with the disease, simply because their cartilage loss has probably been going on for a longer time. So the older you are, the more patient you need to be when it comes to expecting symptomatic relief with these dietary supplements.

Which Supplements You Take. You can't go wrong with either glucosamine or chondroitin sulfate, since the clinical studies involving each of them have produced overwhelmingly positive results. Based on what each supplement does once it gets into the cartilage, it seems likely that they'll have a synergistic effect when taken together, meaning that their combined effect will far outpace what could be achieved by taking either supplement alone. So people who take both supplements are likely to experience benefits sooner than people who take one or the other.

The Doses You Take. As is the case with drugs, the proper dosage of these dietary supplements should be calculated according to your body weight. The more massive you are, the higher the dose that will be needed to reach the joints that are the targets of the treatment. Most of the many clinical trials that have involved glucosamine sulfate have used a dose of 1,500 milligrams per day. With chondroitin sulfate, doses used in clinical studies have ranged between 400 and 1,200 milligrams per day. As a general rule of thumb, those weighing less than 115 pounds should begin supplementing daily with 1,000 milligrams of glucosamine and/or 800 milligrams of chondroitin sulfates; those weighing between 115 and 200 pounds should begin daily supplements of 1,500 milligrams of glucosamine and/or 1,200 milligrams of chondroitin sulfates; and those weighing more than 200 pounds should start supplementing with 2,000 milligrams of glucosamine and/or 1,600 milligrams of chondroitin sulfates daily.

These are *recommended* starting doses only, intended for the "average" person with osteoarthritis. To be on the safe side, you should check with your doctor as to whether these are prudent dosages for you specifically.

Try taking the supplements at the recommended doses for about four weeks. By that time, you should start to notice some positive changes, but it may take longer. Once you start to notice improvement in your symptoms, adjust your dose downward. One tactic is to decrease your daily dosage for each supplement by one capsule every two weeks until you arrive at an effective maintenance level: the lowest daily dose that produces adequate relief from pain and stiffness.

On the other hand, you can go above the starting dosage levels indicated in the table if you feel you need better relief. But do not exceed double the levels listed in the table. For example, if you weigh between 115 and 200 pounds, you probably shouldn't exceed 3,000 milligrams of glucosamine or 2,400 milligrams of chondroitin sulfates a day.

No matter what dose you're taking, cut back on taking the supplements if you think they might be causing complications. Fortunately, clinical studies have shown both glucosamine and chondroitin sulfate to be extremely safe—certainly much safer than the NSAIDs and other drugs commonly used in treating osteoarthritis, which can cause serious damage throughout the body. Among the symptoms that have occasionally been reported by patients taking oral doses of glucosamine and chondroitin sulfate are dyspepsia (heartburn), nausea, stomachache, constipation, and drowsiness.

Rather than swallow your daily dose all at once, divide both supplements into three doses that are taken at intervals throughout the day. Since taking the supplements along with food can minimize any chance of possible stomach upset, it's probably best to take one dose with breakfast, one with lunch, and one with dinner.

What Else You Can Do for Yourself. As we emphasize in *The Arthritis Solution*, the best way to overcome osteoarthritis is to engage in a three-prong offensive. While the dietary supplements glucosamine and chondroitin sulfate are the key prong in that offensive, the other two—a proper diet and adequate exercise—are also important for assuring a successful result. You'll achieve faster results with these dietary supplements if you're also being conscientious about exercising and eating properly.

Supplementing the Supplements

As you'll see in Chapter 8, exercise can help the glucosamine and chondroitin sulfates get to where they need to go. When you swallow them, these nutrients travel to your joints, where they become dissolved in the synovial fluid that surrounds the cartilage. But to put them to work building more cartilage, you've got to get them inside the cartilage, and that's where exercise comes in.

With sufficiently vigorous exercise, you'll be pumping the nutrient-laden synovial fluid throughout the cartilage latticework, so that this fluid lubricates the cartilage and brings the nutrients to the chondrocytes—the all-important cells that take in glucosamine and chondroitin sulfate and use them as the raw material for synthesizing new cartilage. But be careful about doing exercise that's too vigorous, because you might cause further damage to your cartilage—which is the last thing you would want to do.

You can also bolster the effects of glucosamine and chondroitin sulfate through proper diet—and here two key pieces of advice apply: First, if you're overweight, the best way to make sure that these two supplements will work best for you is to slim down. The stress that extra pounds can place on weight-bearing joints, particularly the knees and hips, can squelch whatever benefits these supplements might otherwise offer. Secondly—and no matter how much you weigh—make sure you are consuming the vitamins and minerals that will work together with glucosamine and chondroitin sulfate to help rebuild cartilage. Chapter 7 tells you how to shed those extra pounds and what foods contain the nutrients that are best for your joints.

The Vital Nutrients

It's becoming increasingly clear that glucosamine and chondroitin sulfate aren't the only nutrients you need in order to repair and rebuild cartilage. Several others, particularly certain vitamins, are also crucial for cartilage health. In the following pages, we tell you which ones you can obtain from your diet, and which may require supplements. All are present naturally in many foods, but it is often difficult to obtain optimum amounts from diet alone. Make sure that they're a part of your supplement program, and your joints will be grateful.

Arm Yourself with Antioxidants

There is growing evidence that chemicals called free radicals play a role in causing certain diseases associated with aging, such as cataracts, heart disease, some forms of cancer, and even osteoarthritis. Other chemicals known as antioxidants can act against free radicals and reduce the damage they cause. So there is great hope that these antioxidants (which include vitamins C, E, and beta carotene) may help slow down aging and the diseases that go along with it—including osteoarthritis.

Free radicals are formed constantly within the cells during normal metabolism, when the cells burn oxygen to create energy. The free radicals lack part of their structure and try to regain it by grabbing it from other molecules. This "thievery" by free radicals is the process known as oxidation. As free radicals travel throughout the cell, they disrupt DNA, proteins, and other molecules and generally wreak havoc within the cell. It's this damage that is thought to contribute to aging and to heart disease and other health problems associated with aging. Antioxidants protect these critical cell components from damage by neutralizing the free radicals.

The joints are among the places in the body where free radicals are produced. Indeed, studies have shown that these chemicals damage the key components of cartilage, the proteoglycans and collagen. So could a diet high in antioxidants help to reduce cartilage loss and slow the worsening of osteoarthritis? The first-ever study to address that question was published in 1996 in the journal *Arthritis & Rheumatism*—and the answer was very much in the affirmative.

A Landmark Study

This major finding came out of the famous Framingham Heart Study, in which most of the residents of Framingham, Massachusetts, have been examined every other year for more than forty years. The Framingham study has contributed greatly to the understanding of heart disease—particularly by its discovery that risk factors such as obesity, elevated cholesterol level, and high blood pressure lead to heart disease, the nation's leading killer. But the study has also looked into other health problems, including osteoarthritis.

In this particular study, the Framingham researchers looked for evidence of knee osteoarthritis in 640 people who were evaluated during two exams spaced about ten years apart. Subjects had their knees x-rayed for signs of osteoarthritis, and they also filled out a questionnaire asking about their dietary intake. The researchers used this information to calculate the participants' intake of the antioxidant vitamins C, E, and beta carotene. For each of the three vitamins, all participants were ranked as being either in the bottom third of the whole group in terms of dietary intake, the middle third, or the upper third. The results showed that a diet high in antioxidants, especially vitamin C, was highly beneficial for people with osteoarthritis.

People whose intake of vitamin C was at least 180 milligrams a day were only one-third as likely as those consuming half that amount to have their osteoarthritis worsen over the ten years. This protection was related mainly to reduced cartilage loss. Furthermore, people with osteoarthritis who consumed vitamin C in moderate or high amounts were substantially less likely to develop knee pain.

Some results for vitamin E and beta carotene were also positive, although not quite as impressive as for vitamin C. People consuming the highest amounts of beta carotene had one-half the risk of seeing their osteoarthritis get worse compared with people consuming the least amount of beta carotene. With vitamin E, the beneficial effects were more modest than for the other two antioxidants and were limited to men: Those in the highest category for vitamin E consumption were significantly less likely to have their osteoarthritis worsen compared with men in the lowest category.

"We found that moderate to high antioxidant intake, especially vitamin C, may protect against osteoarthritis progression," the researchers concluded.

The "Big Three" Antioxidants

The findings of the Framingham study support what so much recent research has been suggesting: that consuming adequate amounts of antioxidants can be highly beneficial for people with osteoarthritis. The most important of the antioxidants are the ones scrutinized by the Framingham researchers: vitamin E, vitamin C, and beta carotene. Here's what you need to know about their unique benefits and the supplement levels of each that are likely to be safe as well as effective in keeping your osteoarthritis from progressing.

Vitamin E. Vitamin E is a powerful antioxidant, and more and more studies are indicating its value in combatting disease. In some studies, large numbers of people were asked about their dietary intake of vitamin E and were then followed for several years to see which of them developed certain diseases; in other studies, people were given vitamin E supplements. So far, the evidence suggests that consuming plentiful amounts of vitamin E can offer a cornucopia of benefits.

Vitamin E helps to relieve osteoarthritis, bolster immunity, prevent heart disease, lower the risk of cancers of the colon, rectum, esophagus, and lung, reduce the risk of cataracts, and slow the earlier stages of Parkinson's disease. And most recently, in April of 1997, a study in *The New England Journal of Medicine* reported the exciting news that high doses of vitamin E can slow the progression of Alzheimer's disease.

While it makes sense to include vitamin E-rich foods in your diet (nuts and vegetable oil products are good sources), you'll probably need to take a supplement in order to get the full benefit of vitamin E's antioxidant properties. The most vitamin E that you can expect to derive from a well-balanced diet is about 25 milligrams daily, while studies producing the most encouraging results have typically involved much higher vitamin E intakes—in some cases more than 1,000 milligrams daily. Many top nutritional researchers and public health officials are now convinced vitamin E supplements are useful and are taking the supplements themselves.

The ideal daily dose of vitamin E supplements has not yet been established. The standard recommendation is to stay within the range of 100 International Units (IU) to 400 IU daily, which should provide you with many of vitamin E's benefits, such as protection against heart disease and cancers. But if you're taking vitamin E for your osteoarthritis, you may need higher doses.

In several small studies, patients with osteoarthritis or rheumatoid arthritis took daily doses of up to 1,200 IU of vitamin E. In these studies, it was found that vitamin E relieved pain, swelling, and morning stiffness nearly as effectively as a commonly prescribed anti-inflammatory drug.

Taking vitamin E supplements seems to be a very safe thing to do. One recent review concluded that people can take oral doses of vitamin E of up to 4,500 IU daily without any adverse effects. So far, the one possible downside to taking high doses of vitamin E is that it may increase the risk for hemorrhagic stroke, the less common and more deadly type that is caused by bleeding. On the other hand, for most people that slight mortality risk would be outweighed by vitamin E's help in reducing the risk for both heart disease and thrombotic stroke, the type of stroke caused by blood clots. But anyone already taking anticlotting medications such as warfarin (Coumadin) or ticlopidine (Ticlid) should talk with their doctor before taking vitamin E supplements.

SUPPLEMENTATION RECOMMENDED: Try starting out with a daily supplement dose of 400 IU of vitamin E. If you don't notice improvement after a few weeks, you can increase the dose.

Vitamin C. Thanks to the late Dr. Linus Pauling's tireless promotional efforts, vitamin C is probably the best known of all vitamins. Although this vitamin can't achieve all the wonders that Pauling claimed for it, vitamin C is obviously a key nutrient that offers important health benefits.

Knowledge of vitamin C's benefits dates back to two hundred years ago, when sailors on long voyages died of scurvy, a serious disease in which capillaries hemorrhage because the collagen fibers supporting them have broken down. The British navy found that scurvy could be prevented if the ships were stocked with lemon or lime juice. This action gave British sailors their nickname ("limeys") and eventually led to the discovery of vitamin C, the active ingredient in citrus fruits that was actually protecting the sailors from scurvy.

Today's Recommended Daily Allowance for vitamin C is pegged at 60 milligrams a day (100 milligrams for smokers), the amount sufficient to ward off scurvy. But there's growing evidence that much higher amounts of vitamin C improve health in other ways. These health benefits relate to vitamin C's role as an antioxidant—an effect that may offer protection against heart disease and cancer, the nation's two leading killers, and also against osteoarthritis.

Studies have shown that people with high vitamin C levels in their blood tend to have more high-density lipoprotein cholesterol—the "good" cholesterol that lowers heart disease risk—than do people with low blood levels of vitamin C. Furthermore, the artery-clogging "bad" cholesterol, or low-density lipoprotein cholesterol, only appears to clog arteries when it has been damaged, or oxidized, by free radicals. Studies show that vitamin C surrounds LDL molecules in the blood and protects them from becoming oxidized. Vitamin C's probable benefit against heart disease is underlined by several population studies that have found a lower rate of heart disease among people who consume the most vitamin C.

The same free radicals that damage LDL cholesterol can also damage the cells of the body, causing them to multiply out of control and become cancerous. Vitamin C may help to combat cancer in two ways: by neutralizing free radicals and also by boosting the body's immune defenses. Several population studies have found a link between high levels of vitamin C consumption and lower rates of cancer, especially cancers all along the digestive tract—of the mouth, throat, stomach, colon, and rectum.

When it comes to helping combat osteoarthritis, vitamin C's antioxidant powers also come into play. As noted earlier, it's now known that free radicals are produced within the joints—and of all the antioxidants, vitamin C may have the best chance of reaching those free radicals and neutralizing them before they can cause damage.

Vitamin C is a water-soluble vitamin rather than a fat-soluble molecule like the other two major antioxidant vitamins, beta carotene and vitamin E. Since the joints are awash in synovial fluid, which is largely water, water-soluble vitamin C would have the best chance of getting into the synovial fluid and doing battle with the free radicals. (Recall that in the Framingham study, described earlier in this chapter, vitamin C appeared to be the most useful antioxidant against osteoarthritis.)

It's also quite possible that vitamin C helps against osteoarthritis through its more traditional role in the body: maintaining and building collagen, the structural fibers found in many tissues of the body, including cartilage. It's known that production of type II collagen—the main type found in cartilage—depends on the presence of vitamin C.

Studies in animals have shown that too little vitamin C shuts down not only cartilage's collagen production but also its output of proteoglycans, the other main component of cartilage. This means that vitamin C probably helps to augment the dietary supplements glucosamine and chondroitin sulfate in their crucial task of bolstering the number of proteoglycans in cartilage.

How much vitamin C should you get every day? If you consume a healthy diet emphasizing fruits and vegetables, you could certainly take in 500 milligrams of vitamin C a day, which easily exceeds the Recommended Dietary Allowance of 60 milligrams. That's even well above the 200-milligram level that some experts are now recommending as a better RDA for vitamin C. But for some people, vitamin C supplements may be a good idea.

Unfortunately, many people fall short of consuming enough of the fruits and vegetables that can provide adequate amounts of vitamin C. Others, such as the elderly, don't absorb vitamins and other nutrients very efficiently. And still others, such as adolescents and pregnant women, have high nutritional demands that may require supplementation not only with vitamin C but with other vitamins as well. If your vitamin C intake is inadequate or if you just want to be prudent, then vitamin C supplements or a multivitamin containing C may be the way to go for protecting your joints.

It's probably not a good idea to go beyond vitamin C supplementation of 1,000 mg per day. At doses higher than that, vitamin C can cause nausea, abdominal pain, and diarrhea, although those complications are rare. People who probably have the greatest need for taking vitamin C supplements are the elderly (the ability to absorb vitamins declines in older people) and adolescents and pregnant women, whose bodies have particularly high metabolic needs for vitamin C that their diets might not be able to satisfy.

SUPPLEMENTATION RECOMMENDED: If you don't eat five servings of fruits and vegetables a day, take a daily vitamin C supplement of 200 mg.

Beta Carotene. Until 1994 beta carotene was the hottest supplement around, mainly because it was thought to be the nutrient that was best at protecting against cancer. But around that time two well-designed clinical trials found that beta carotene supplements may actually increase the risk of lung cancer in smokers, and one of the studies found a possibly increased risk of heart disease as well. A third beta carotene study, lasting longer than the other two, found no increased cancer risk for nonsmokers—but neither did it find any benefit.

As a result of these recent findings, most nutrition experts now recommend against taking beta carotene supplements. But consuming beta catotene in more moderate amounts, through your diet, is still an excellent idea—for help against osteoarthritis as well as for your overall health.

Beta carotene is one member of a large family of substances known as carotenoids, which are found mainly in fruits and vegetables. The body converts beta carotene and many of its brethren carotenoids into vitamin A. Beta carotene has captured the spotlight simply because it's the most plentiful carotenoid and the one that's most readily convertible to vitamin A.

The many studies that have found lower rates of cancer and other benefits from beta carotene—including the Framingham study, which found beta carotene had a protective effect against osteoarthritis—have all involved people whose *diets* included plenty of fruits and vegetables that were rich in beta carotene. And none of these studies found that diets rich in beta carotene were associated with an increased cancer risk.

This may explain why beta carotene supplements showed little benefit in the recent clinical trials. The useful ingredient in foods rich in beta carotene may not be beta carotene at all but rather one or more of the many other carotenoids or other nutrients present in these foods. That's why getting beta carotene from your diet rather than from a supplement may be especially important, since it means you'll also be consuming other carotenoids that may actually be responsible for the health benefits from beta carotene-rich foods.

SUPPLEMENTATION NOT RECOMMENDED: The strongest evidence for protection lies not with beta carotene supplements but with carotene-rich fruits and vegetables. Luckily, it's very easy to obtain plenty of beta carotene from a healthy diet that features a variety of fruits and vegetables. In Chapter 7, we list numerous produce items and the beta carotene content of each.

"D" for Defense Against Osteoarthritis

When vitamin D comes to mind, you probably think of bones. The normal metabolism of bone—the building up and breaking down of bone that occurs all the time—depends on getting enough of this vitamin, which helps the body absorb calcium. But since bone and cartilage are so intimately connected, it makes sense that vitamin D could have an influence on osteoarthritis as well.

Some researchers have speculated that bone "quality" and the way bone reacts to weight-bearing activities and other stresses could influence whether osteoarthritis remains stable or gets worse. In other words, when people have "soft" bones—perhaps because of inadequate vitamin D intake—osteoarthritis may be a more serious problem. Even more pertinent, research has found that vitamin D seems to have a direct effect on the cartilage of the joints, by stimulating cartilage cells to produce proteoglycans, a key component of cartilage. So researchers in Boston decided to see if the amount of vitamin D in the diets might have an influence on osteoarthritis.

This vitamin D study was yet another offshoot of the Framingham study, which we described earlier in this chapter when discussing the antioxidants. As with the study involving the antioxidants, the vitamin D study involved examining residents of Framingham, Massachusetts, for evidence of osteoarthritis of the knee, assessing their dietary vitamin intake, and then looking for connections between vitamin intake and their risk for developing osteoarthritis or having their osteoarthritis get worse over the next ten years.

In addition to the vitamin D we get from food, we also synthesize our own vitamin D when we're exposed to sunlight. So in this study, the researchers looked not only at the amount of vitamin D in people's diets but also—to get a more complete idea of vitamin D's presence—measured the level of vitamin D in their serum. The results, published in 1996 in the *Annals of Internal Medicine*, showed that vitamin D does have an important influence on osteoarthritis.

To quote the researchers: "Our study suggests that persons with low intake and low serum levels of vitamin D are approximately three times more likely to have progression of established osteoarthritis of the knee than are persons with high intake and high serum levels." The researchers also noted that low serum levels of vitamin D were associated with a loss of cartilage in the knee joint.

If you have osteoarthritis, you should certainly make sure that you're consuming the Recommended Dietary Allowance of vitamin D each day, which is 400 International Units. You can do three things to get more vitamin D in your body: Get outside more so you get more sun exposure, consume more dairy products, or take vitamin D supplements.

If you opt for vitamin D supplements, you need to

be cautious because vitamin D is a fat-soluble vitamin that is not excreted readily, so it can rather easily build up to toxic levels in your tissues. Too much of it can cause calcium deposits in the body, leading to serious damage to the kidneys and the cardiovascular system.

The level at which vitamin D causes harm may in some cases be only five times the Recommended Dietary Allowance for vitamin D. So to be on the safe side, stay away from single-nutrient vitamin D supplements. If you happen to be consuming a couple of glasses of vitamin D-fortified milk a day, taking vitamin D supplements could actually tip your vitamin D intake into the danger zone.

SUPPLEMENTATION NOT RECOMMENDED: Instead of taking a vitamin D supplement, try to satisfy your vitamin D needs by consuming low-fat dairy products. Alternatively, take a multivitamin containing 400 IU of vitamin D, the Recommended Dietary Allowance. That's the amount you'd obtain by drinking a quart of milk.

Folate and Vitamin B_{12}

A recent study carried out at the University of Missouri-Columbia indicates these two B vitamins can work in tandem against osteoarthritis. Researchers there gave supplements of folate (6,400 micrograms per day) and B_{12} (20 micrograms per day) to men and women with osteoarthritis of the hands. After two months, the people who took the supplements had fewer tender hand joints than a group who took NSAIDs instead of the vitamins.

Most of the vitamin B_{12} in the human diet comes from meat and dairy products. But to obtain the 20 micrograms of B_{12} per day used in the University of Missouri study, you can't rely on food but will have to get your vitamin B_{12} from supplements.

SUPPLEMENTATION RECOMMENDED: Too much vitamin B_{12} can cause toxicity, but intakes up to 100 micrograms per day are considered safe.

Besides its apparent usefulness against osteoarthritis, folate—also known as folic acid—plays several crucial roles in maintaining good health. If women's diets are deficient in folate during the early weeks of pregnancy, their babies are at risk for developing spina bifida, a serious congenital disease in which the spinal cord is not completely formed. Folate also reduces levels of an amino acid in the blood called homocysteine. Elevated levels of homocysteine are believed to damage the lining of blood vessel walls and contribute to heart disease.

Folic acid is found in green leafy vegetables such as brussels sprouts, lettuce, and spinach and in many fruits, including apples and oranges. By 1998, the FDA will require that all enriched grain products such as bread, pasta, rice, flour, and corn meal be fortified with folic acid. The current Recommended Dietary Allowance for folate is 200 micrograms per day, although many experts believe that level should be raised to 400 micrograms per day.

SUPPLEMENTATION RECOMMENDED: Most multiple-vitamin preparations contain folate, and you can also buy it as a single-nutrient supplement. Taking supplements to attain the megadose of folate used in the University of Missouri study—6,400 micrograms per day—is probably safe, but you should consult your physician before taking that high a daily dosage of this vitamin.

Fish Oil

In the past few years, fish oil supplements have attracted interest because they may play a role in fighting arthritis. These oils, obtained mainly from cold-water fish, are rich in omega-3 fatty acids. Only recently have omega-3 fatty acids been recognized as being crucial to the normal functioning of the body.

When ingested, omega-3 fatty acids have the ability to decrease inflammation—making fish oils potentially useful for people with rheumatoid arthritis, in which inflammation is a significant problem. Indeed, several controlled studies, most of them using high doses of fish oil, have found that some patients with rheumatoid arthritis do experience improvement in tender joints from the use of fish oil. The clinical benefits are usually modest, and people must take fish oil daily for at least six months before noticeable improvement occurs.

Fish oil is primarily marketed as eicosapentaenoic acid (EPA), the predominant omega-3 fatty acid in fish. Fish oil capsules are sold in health food stores under a number of brands, including MaxEPA, SuperEPA, and Cardi-Omega 3. Another type of omega-3 fatty acid found in fish oil is docosahexaenoic acid (DHA).

A 1993 review of fish oil use in the treatment of arthritis, published in the *British Journal of Rheumatology*, concluded that "work to date on fish oils for rheumatoid arthritis patients is interesting and promising and treatment appears to be safe." But much less research has been done on whether fish oil can help against osteoarthritis. In the one controlled study carried out on fish oil for the treatment of osteoarthritis, twenty-six patients were given either EPA or a placebo oil for six months. Afterward, the patients taking EPA experienced somewhat less pain and less interference with daily activities than patients in the placebo group. Although the differences between the two groups were not significant, the authors concluded that their results were sufficiently promising to justify a full-scale trial, involving larger numbers of people, to find out more about fish oil and its possible usefulness against osteoarthritis. That study has yet to be done.

SUPPLEMENTATION NOT RECOMMENDED: People taking fish oil supplements in clinical trials have generally consumed 4 to 6 grams of fish oil daily. That can be expensive (up to forty dollars a week) and may not be good for your overall health. The supplements are basically fish fat, and taking them in high doses may actually increase your level of LDL cholesterol, the bad kind that's associated with artery clogging. Even with more moderate doses, fish oil pills can cause digestive upsets including diarrhea, upset stomach, and burping, and can also leave users smelling fishy.

Osteoarthritis and Hormone Replacement Therapy

Hormone replacement therapy isn't something that normally comes to mind as a treatment for osteoarthritis. But recent research indicates that it may help prevent older women from developing the disease.

Each year, thousands of women who reach menopause take supplemental hormones—estrogen and often progesterone—to replace the estrogen that they stop producing at that time. A prime reason for taking estrogen is to relieve some of the unpleasant symptoms of menopause, such as hot flashes, mood swings, and vaginal dryness. In addition, taking estrogen at menopause helps protect women from two serious health problems that become particularly common after menopause: heart disease and the bone-thinning disorder osteoporosis. Several studies have suggested that supplemental estrogen may also protect women from developing osteoarthritis in the knees and hips.

In one study, Boston University researchers followed 557 women between the ages of sixty-three and ninety-two who were participating in the long-running Framingham Heart Study. The researchers found that osteoarthritis of the knee affected twenty percent of the women who had not had hormone replacement therapy, 17.8 percent of the women who had been given hormone therapy for one to five years, and only 12.7 percent of women who had used hormone replacement for more than five years.

In addition, the researchers found that osteoarthritis was least likely to occur in women who were currently using replacement hormones. Their overall conclusion was that hormone therapy helps to prevent osteoarthritis from developing and progressing in older women.

Hormone replacement therapy is not a treatment that women should undertake lightly. While it offers women undeniable benefits, it may pose risks as well. In particular, some studies suggest that women who use replacement hormones may face an increased risk of breast cancer. Hormone replacement therapy's possible protective effect against osteoarthritis is one more thing for women to consider when deciding whether to choose it.

Chapter 6

Questions and Answers about Supplements

In this chapter, we answer some of the questions that may have arisen as you've been reading about glucosamine and chondroitin sulfate.

Q: The clinical studies on glucosamine and chondroitin sulfate that you've described are impressive, but I'd feel more comfortable taking these supplements if I knew of some actual people who'd gotten better after using them. Can you name any?

A: We can tell you about improvements not only in people but in their pets. A well-known recent convert to glucosamine and chondroitin sulfate is Jane E. Brody, science writer and health columnist for the *New York Times*. In the newspaper's January 15, 1997 issue, Brody wrote about improvements in her osteoarthritic knees that she attributed to the supplements:

"The [combination glucosamine and chondroitin sulfate] product had seemed to be so effective in countering the arthritic lameness of my eleven-year-old spaniel that I decided to try it myself. After two months on this remedy, I am about thirty percent better. I am not pain-free and I still tend to get a little stiff after prolonged sitting, but I have stopped limping, I am playing tennis and ice skating with less pain, and my knees have stopped swelling after strenuous activity."

Another believer, a prominent orthopedic surgeon, was interviewed in the April 9, 1997 issue of the Boston *Globe* by science writer Judy Foreman. Dr. David Hungerford, chief of orthopedics at the Good Samaritan Hospital in Baltimore, was described as being eager to conduct a clinical study on the supplements. "But meanwhile," according to the article, "this Johns Hopkins surgeon whose arthritic hands perform three hundred joint replacement operations a year, many on people with arthritic knees, has begun taking the stuff himself."

"I've had significant improvement," he says.

The next person interviewed in the article was Dr. Joseph B. Houpt, director of rheumatology at Mt. Sinai Hospital in Toronto. Houpt, the article stated, "is already doing a study [of the supplement glucosamine], prompted by enthusiastic reports from patients who buy the remedy in health food stores. And by watching his dog."

"I have two yellow Labs," he says. "One was creaking and groaning, unable to jump over stumps, unable to jump up on the couch. She's like a pup since taking the drug."

Q: I can't find chondroitin sulfate supplements in my health food store. But the manager says that other supplements he carries—mucopolysaccharide complexes, shark cartilage, and bovine cartilage—can provide the same benefits. Is he right?

A: That depends. Chondroitin sulfate is not made in the laboratory but instead comes from animal cartilage—most commonly shark cartilage and the tracheas of cows (bovine cartilage). When you buy supplements of shark or bovine cartilage, you'll be getting some chondroitin sulfate but perhaps not too much.

Chondroitin sulfate is just one member of a family of compounds called mucopolysaccharides—which themselves are but one part of cartilage. Shark or bovine cartilage supplements typically will consist of about fifteen percent chondroitin sulfate; the products sold as mucopolysaccharide complexes should be somewhat richer in chondroitin sulfate.

By contrast, products labeled as chondroitin sulfate, or as bovine or shark cartilage *extract*, have been processed and purified so that they should contain a much higher percentage of chondroitin sulfate—up to ninety percent in some cases. For example, Vitamin Research Products sells a product called Bovine Cartilage Extract; each 550-milligram capsule of Bovine Cartilage Extract is said to provide 500 milligrams of chondroitin sulfate. (See table on page 76 for more information on this and other chondroitin sulfate and glucosamine products.)

Q: My health food store carries a supplement called n-acetyl glucosamine, referred to as NAG. Product literature for NAG claims that it's superior to glucosamine sulfate—better absorbed and more efficiently utilized in the body. Should I choose it over glucosamine sulfate for my osteoarthritis?

A: Actually, n-acetyl glucosamine may not work quite as well as some of the other types of glucosamine.

When you start reading the labels of glucosamine products, you'll see that there are many varieties now being offered: glucosamine sulfate, glucosamine hydrochloride (also known as glucosamine HCl), n-acetyl glucosamine, glucosamine chlorohydrate (which is the same as glucosamine HCl), D-glucosamine, glucosamine hydroiodide, and glucosamine with potassium chloride added. All the clinical studies that have been published on glucosamine have used just one form of it—glucosamine sulfate (although glucosamine HCl has achieved good results in animal studies, and it is the form of glucosamine being used in clinical studies on osteoarthritis now underway in the U.S.).

In one laboratory study, researchers took various forms of glucosamine and "fed" them to cartilage cells in a petri dish. They then compared the different forms of glucosamine: How effective were they at stimulating the cartilage cells to produce one of the components of cartilage known as mucopolysaccharides? Of the different types studied, the researchers found that glucosamine sulfate and glucosamine hydrochloride did equally well in stimulating cartilage production. But by comparison, they found that n-acetylglucosamine "caused a considerably smaller increase" in cartilage.

As you'll note in the table beginning on page 76 in Chapter 5, glucosamine sulfate and glucosamine HCl are the types of glucosamine most often used in glucosamine products. Milligram for milligram, they should work equally well in your body to restore cartilage. But with glucosamine HCl, you'll be getting slightly more bang for your buck. That's because a 500-milligram capsule of glucosamine HCl, for example, will contain slightly more of the active ingredient—glucosamine—than will a 500-milligram capsule of glucosamine sulfate.

One caution: People with thyroid problems should probably avoid glucosamine hydroiodide, since it could alter their thyroid function.

Q: Where does glucosamine come from?

A: Glucosamine is made from crab shell, and the main source of it in the U.S. is Alaska king crab. First the shells are cleaned and pulverized into a powder. Then a chemical called chitin—a polysaccharide that is an important component of shells—is extracted. The chitin is then processed further to obtain glucosamine. Whether the final product is glucosamine sulfate, glucosamine HCl, or some other type depends on the chemical process used.

Q: When discussing the clinical research on glucosamine, you mention a European study in which patients were given glucosamine injections. Are glucosamine injections available in this country, and is there any advantage to taking glucosamine this way?

A: Both oral and injectible forms of glucosamine have been used for years in Europe, while only the oral form is available in this country.

When most anything is swallowed, some of it will be digested before it can be absorbed into the bloodstream. Giving glucosamine by injection means you are bypassing the gastrointestinal tract and maximizing the amount that gets into the bloodstream. However, oral glucosamine is very well absorbed, with studies showing that about ninety percent of what you swallow enters the bloodstream. So the advantage of the injections isn't all that great.

Q: When I buy supplements containing glucosamine or chondroitin sulfate, do I have any assurance that the capsules really do contain the active ingredient and in the quantities claimed on the label?

A: Compared with drugs, the manufacture of dietary supplements, such as glucosamine and chondroitin sulfate receives scant attention from the Food and Drug Administration. For example, FDA inspectors don't do what they do at the country's drug manufacturing facilities, which is to keep an eye on quality control and check records to make sure that the proper ingredients are being used in every batch of the product. Nevertheless, some supplement makers have their own production and quality control standards that rival those used by the pharmaceutical companies. Some companies, for example, test every batch of a supplement they make, to assure that products are free of impurities and contain the correct amounts of the active ingredients.

If you're curious about the way a supplement is made, write or call the manufacturer and ask for information on the testing and other quality control procedures. In particular, you should ask if the company meets FDA standards for making food products. Companies that devote a lot of attention to quality are usually happy to tell you how their products are made. The product table in Chapter 4 lists the toll-free numbers for many supplement makers.

Q: My doctor has given me the go-ahead to try glucosamine and chondroitin sulfate for my osteoarthritis, but he says I'll probably have to pay for it out of my own pocket. Is he right?

A: Unfortunately, yes. Since both products are dietary supplements and not drugs, they are not covered by most health insurance policies.

Q: I've been taking a product that combines glucosamine and chondroitin sulfate in the same capsule. Is there any particular advantage to taking a combination capsule, and why do they also contain a small amount of ascorbate (vitamin C) and manganese?

A: Aside from convenience and perhaps price, taking a combination capsule probably offers no particular advantage over taking the glucosamine and chondroitin sulfates separately.

Manganese is commonly added to capsules of glucosamine and/or chondroitin sulfate because this mineral stimulates cartilage to produce one of its two key building blocks, molecules called proteoglycans. Glucosamine and chondroitin sulfate serve as raw materials in the manufacture of these proteoglycans. Vitamin C enhances any dietary supplement's absorption into the bloodstream. It's also an especially useful companion for these supplements because vitamin C helps to maintain and build collagen, the structural fibers that are a major component of cartilage.

Q: I'm on a tight budget and may have to choose between buying glucosamine and chondroitin sulfate for treating my osteoarthritis. Since I'll be choosing just one, which of the two would you recommend?

A: Go for the glucosamine. For one thing, you'll probably be getting a bigger bang for your buck. That's because glucosamine is a tiny molecule that's efficiently absorbed into your bloodstream after you swallow it. Chondroitin sulfate, on the other hand, consists of huge "macromolecules" that are not absorbed as efficiently as glucosamine.

Furthermore, if you look at the clinical studies that have been done, glucosamine sulfate has the edge in terms of the number of impressive studies carried out on patients with osteoarthritis. It has been found to offer major benefits, not only in relieving symptoms but in actually healing damaged cartilage. Although chondroitin sulfate has not been involved in as many studies, those that have been carried out certainly indicate that it's effective.

Q: How much will it cost for me to take both glucosamine and chondroitin sulfates for my osteoarthritis?

A: That will vary, depending most crucially on where you buy your supplements and what your daily dose is. But on average, taking a daily dose of both supplements will cost between fifty and one hundred dollars per month. That may sound steep, but it's less than the monthly cost of many prescription-strength pain relievers—and the supplements are certainly much safer.

Q: Is there anything I can do to lower the cost?

A: You can do several things to reduce the cost of taking these supplements, including:

Buy the large size. You can almost always save money by purchasing the manufacturer's biggest bottle.

Take the lowest dose necessary. See the recommendations on page 91 for a suggested "starting dose" for glucosamine and chondroitin sulfate based upon your weight.

Reduce your dosage when you notice improvement. You will—we hope—notice an improvement in your symptoms after several weeks, and at that point you should begin slowly cutting back on your intake, perhaps by one capsule per week for each supplement. Some people have been able to cut their initial dose by half or even by two-thirds and still experience the benefits these supplements offer.

Let the pain and stiffness in your joints be your guide as you adjust the dosage. You may find that you can maintain the good feeling in your joints for considerably less money than when you first started taking the supplements.

Employ the two other prongs of our three-prong attack. Glucosamine and chondroitin sulfate are the most promising products to come along in many years for treating osteoarthritis, and they're the focus of this book. But as you'll see, *The Arthritis Solution* also stresses the need to eat right and to exercise regularly if you're to combat osteoarthritis successfully on all fronts. Proper diet and exercise can truly "supplement the supplements," making them work more effectively and, ultimately, allowing you to cut back on the number of capsules or tablets that you need to take.

Q: Will I have to take these supplements indefinitely?

A: Since osteoarthritis is a chronic condition, you should view the supplement treatment—or any other osteoarthritis therapy, for that matter—as long-term maintenance therapy, similar to controlling hypertension with diuretics or diabetes with insulin. But as we've noted in *The Arthritis Solution*, these two supplements appear to do more than just soothe symptoms and keep osteoarthritis stabilized. There is evidence that they also help to rebuild cartilage, so you may find you can taper off the supplements completely—for months or even years.

Q: Is it all right to take glucosamine and chondroitin sulfate along with the pain relievers I've been prescribed for my osteoarthritis?

A: There is no evidence to suggest that either of these supplements interferes with osteoarthritis drugs or vice versa. One benefit to taking the supplements is that they may allow you to cut back on the dosage of pain-relieving drugs that you need. But be sure to consult with your doctor before changing your dosage.

Q: Is there any osteoarthritis patient who probably won't gain much benefit from using glucosamine and/or chondroitin sulfate?

A: Those troubled by severe osteoarthritis, in which the cartilage in a joint has virtually disappeared, probably shouldn't expect much benefit. The reason: These supplements work primarily by stimulating the cartilage cells, known as chondrocytes, to get busy building more cartilage. But if there is little or no cartilage in the joint to begin with, there is not much the supplements can do to improve things.

Q: I've only heard about the usefulness of glucosamine and chondroitin sulfate for treating osteoarthritis. Have any studies looked into whether these supplements might have beneficial effects against rheumatoid arthritis?

A: There has been some preliminary work in this area.

Up until recently, studies involving these two dietary supplements have been aimed at treating osteoarthritis, and for good reason. Osteoarthritis involves cartilage—specifically, an imblance between cartilage synthesis and cartilage breakdown within the joint. Over the years, if the breakdown of cartilage occurs faster than it can be made, the net result is osteoarthritis, the wearing away of cartilage. Glucosamine and chondroitin sulfates can intervene against osteoarthritis by stimulating cartilage production and inhibiting cartilage breakdown.

By contrast, the damage to cartilage and other joint tissues that occurs in rheumatoid arthritis is due almost entirely to the destructive impact of inflammation. Glucosamine and chondroitin sulfate do have some antiinflammatory effect, but this effect wasn't considered potent enough to have much impact against rheumatoid arthritis. Recent evidence, however, suggests that using the two supplements in combination may offer some help against types of arthritis that are autoimmune in nature, which would include rheumatoid arthritis.

At the North American Veterinary Conference in January 1997, researchers from Johns Hopkins University School of Medicine announced results of a study involving two groups of rats. One group was fed a combination glucosamine/chondroitin sulfate product for ten days, while the other group—the control group—did not receive the supplements. All the rats were then injected with a protein that causes rats to develop a form of autoimmune arthritis.

Twenty-two of twenty-three rats in the control group developed the autoimmune arthritis (96 percent of animals) versus only thirteen of twenty-four rats that received the combination glucosamine/chondroitin sulfate product (54 percent of animals)—a statistically significant difference.

The researchers said their study had been inspired by anecdotal reports that children with juvenile rheumatoid arthritis—as well as animals with autoimmune degenerative joint disease—experience pain reduction and improved range of motion with a combination glucosamine/chondroitin sulfate product.

This preliminary animal study is promising, but much more work needs to be done before glucosamine and chondroitin sulfate can be recommended for rheumatoid arthritis or other forms of autoimmune arthritis.

Q: I'm forty-five years old, and although I don't have osteoarthritis yet, it's clear from the demographics of this disease that I've got a better than even chance of developing it by the time I'm sixty-five. Should I consider taking these supplements as a preventive measure?

A: X-ray studies have shown that osteoarthritis is an insidious process that usually begins long before people become aware of it. According to these studies, joints typically have X-ray evidence of cartilage loss several years before patients begin complaining of pain and stiffness.

Many of the supplements people take are for preventive purposes—vitamin E to prevent heart disease and several types of cancer, vitamin C to ward off colds, etc. So if you think you're at risk for a slowly developing disease like osteoarthritis, it probably makes sense to consider taking glucosamine and chondroitin sulfate even if your joints have not yet started to act up.

Chapter 7

Eat to Beat Osteoarthritis

What you eat and how much you eat can profoundly affect whether your osteoarthritis improves or worsens. It can even influence whether you develop the disease in the first place.

As we've seen, two nutritional supplements, chondroitin sulfate and glucosamine, can help you rebuild cartilage that has been lost through osteoarthritis. This chapter will show you how the nutrients in the foods you eat, including vitamins such as C and E, can also contribute to this rebuilding process. But the success of all these nutrients depends to a large extent on your *total* diet: If you've put on some extra pounds, the additional stress they're putting on your joints can overwhelm whatever benefits you may gain from the supplements.

The Many Reasons for Losing Weight

Being overweight is now recognized as a major cause of osteoarthritis, particularly osteoarthritis of the knee and hip. Shedding some pounds if you're overweight may be one of the most important things you can do for your joints. And as we'll see, you'll almost always have to combine diet with exercise if you want to keep those lost pounds from coming back.

Carrying around extra pounds will definitely aggravate your joint problems—which makes perfect sense when you think about it. If you had a sore knee, wouldn't you hate the thought of walking around all day carrying a forty-pound suitcase? As far as your knee is concerned, forty extra pounds on your frame exerts the same amount of pressure and pain as that heavy suitcase. Fortunately, even a modest weight loss of a few pounds can make your joints feel dramatically better.

In addition to easing osteoarthritis pain, losing weight can help you do something else that may be even more important: Weight loss can actually keep your unaffected joints from developing the disease.

The role of weight loss in preventing osteoarthritis in overweight people was first demonstrated in 1992—the first study ever to show that osteoarthritis was potentially preventable. Writing in the *Annals of Internal Medicine*, researchers found that overweight women, middle-aged and older, can significantly reduce their risk for developing osteoarthritis of the knee by losing weight. And the weight loss didn't have to be drastic. By losing just eleven pounds over a ten-year period, the study concluded, an overweight woman could reduce her risk for developing knee osteoarthritis by fifty percent.

In addition to benefiting your joints, losing weight can reduce your risk for developing a slew of other serious health problems including high blood pressure, an elevated blood cholesterol level, heart disease, several types of cancer, gallstones, low-back problems, and sleep disorders.

Of course, some people seem to have a strong genetic predisposition toward being obese, and for them, losing weight is nearly impossible. Recent studies suggest an explanation: A genetic defect has been found that makes some people burn calories abnormally slowly. But the vast majority of people have genes that permit a wide range of possible weights—and whether they end up at the high end or the low end of that spectrum depends largely on what they do, or don't do. For example, studies of identical twins, who are exactly the same genetically, have found that one twin may be obese while the other one isn't—meaning that their weight differences are due to their health habits and not their genes.

Are You Overweight?

For most of us, determining whether we're overweight is painfully simple—a glance in the mirror will usually suffice. But more scientific methods are also available, including the height and weight table below. If you've "grown beyond" the recommended weight range for your height, it's probably time to develop a plan of action.

An even better measure of your risk for osteoarthritis and other health problems is the Body Mass Index, a ratio calculated from your weight and your height. For the address of an Internet web site that can make this calculation for you, see "Resources."

Cut Back on Fat

If you are overweight, obviously one of the most important changes you can make in your diet is to eat

Healthy Weight Ranges for Both Men and Women

Height (without shoes)	Weight (without clothes)
4'10"	91–119 pounds
4'11"	94–124
5'0"	97–128
5'1"	101–132
5'2"	104–137
5'3"	107–141
5'4"	111–146
5'5"	114–150
5'6"	118–155
5'7"	121–160
5'8"	125–164
5'9"	129–169
5'10"	132–174
5'11"	136–179
6'0"	140–184
6'1"	144–189
6'2"	148–195
6'3"	152–200
6'4"	156–205
6'5"	160–211
6'6"	164–216

SOURCE: U.S. Dietary Guidelines for Americans, 1995

less fat. Gram for gram, fat contains more than twice as many calories as protein or carbohydrate (nine calories are in a gram of fat versus four in a gram of protein or carbohydrate). Furthermore, the calories from fat apparently are more readily stored as fat on the body than are calories from carbohydrates or protein.

Although we definitely eat too much fat, as a nation we've actually done better in recent years. For example, over the past quarter century, we've pared our consumption of red meat by more than ten percent in favor of leaner foods such as chicken, turkey, and fish, and we've reduced our thirst for whole milk by more than forty percent, turning instead to low-fat or skim milk. Yet during the same period, the percentage of total calories that we derive from fat has decreased only modestly—from forty-one percent to about thirty-six percent.

The problem is this: While we Americans have curbed our appetite for traditional sources of fat, we have sharply increased our intake of "invisible" fats—mainly vegetable fats—in baked goods, fast foods, salad dressings, and other processed foods.

The following table shows that making some minor substitutions among the foods you buy can have a major impact on fat and the calories you consume from fat. Consider just one example: Pretzels and potato chips are both salty snacks—but the resemblance ends there. More than one-third by weight of a potato chip is "invisible" fat. One ounce of potato chips contains thirteen times as much total fat as is contained in one ounce of twist pretzels.

Also listed in the table is the percentage of calories from fat for each food. Federal recommendations suggest that, on average, people restrict the percentage of their calories from fat to thirty percent. And many scientists believe that fat intake ideally should be much lower, with no more than fifteen or twenty percent of calories from fat.

Watch Out for Low-Fat Calories

While you're monitoring your fat consumption, don't become so preoccupied that you neglect calories from other sources. On average, Americans have actually reduced their fat intake by a modest amount over the past decade, yet they've still gotten significantly heavier. A federal survey released early in 1997 found that the percentage of overweight children, teenagers, and adults in the U.S. is "at an all-time high." Among adults, some thirty-three percent of men and thirty-six percent of women now qualify as being overweight. The likely explanation: While we're eating less fat, our total caloric intake has actually increased, thanks to the lure of "low-fat" and "no-fat" food.

Many people mistakenly assume that they don't need to show restraint when eating food labeled as low-fat or fat-free. However, many low-fat foods actually contain as many or even *more* calories than their regular versions, since manufacturers must compensate for the fat they've removed from the food—and they do so by adding a whole lot of sugar. To make sure you reduce both calories and fat in your diet, you should cut back on both fatty foods and calorie-rich low-fat foods. This, of course, is the essence of a good diet—but even that probably won't be enough to rid you of pounds.

The problem, as recent studies have shown, is that the body reacts to dieting as it would to starvation: by slowing down its metabolic rate. To make matters worse, much of the weight you lose by going on a stringent low-calorie diet comes not from fat but from muscle tissue, exactly the kind of tissue that you *don't* want to lose.

Losing muscle cuts into your strength, which isn't good. And it also slows down your metabolic rate— the rate at which you burn calories when not exercising. Since muscle is a high-calorie-burning tissue, losing some of it means you're now burning off fewer calories than before. This explains why losing more

Fats in Food

Foods		Total fat in grams	Calories	% cal from fat
Tuna	Chicken of the Sea chunk light in water, 3 oz., undrained	1.0	89	10
	Chicken of the Sea chunk light in vegetable oil, 3 oz., undrained	17.6	254	62
Chicken	Roasted light meat, no skin, 3.5 oz.	4.5	171	24
	Fried, battered, light meat, with skin, 3.5 oz.	15.3	274	50
Turkey	Roasted, light meat, no skin, 3.5 oz.	2.9	152	17
	Roasted, light meat, w/skin, 3.5 oz.	7.6	189	36
Cold cuts	Ham, 3 slices, 3 oz.	9.0	156	52
	Beef salami, 3 slices, 2.4 oz.	13.7	174	71
	Beef bologna, 3 slices, 2.4 oz.	19.3	216	80
Meat	Veal cutlet, leg, breaded/pan-fried, 3 oz.	5.3	175	27
	Sirloin steak, lean only, broiled, 3 oz.	7.7	180	39
	Sirloin steak, lean & fat, broiled, 3 oz.	15.7	240	59
	Bacon, cooked, 3 medium slices	9.0	109	74

Category	Food			
Milk	Skim milk, 1 cup	0.4	86	4
	Buttermilk, 1 cup	2.2	99	20
	Low-fat (1% fat), 1 cup	2.6	102	23
	Whole milk (3.3% fat), 1 cup	8.1	150	49
Cheese	Cottage cheese, low-fat (1%), 4 oz.	1.2	82	13
	Cottage cheese, creamed, 4 oz.	5.1	117	39
	Swiss cheese, 1 oz.	7.8	107	66
	Processed American cheese, 1 oz.	9.9	99	90
Yogurt	Yogurt, skim-milk plain, 8 oz.	0.4	127	3
	Yogurt, whole-milk plain, 8 oz.	7.4	139	48
Ice Cream	Light n' Lively vanilla-flavored premium ice milk, 4 fl. oz.	2.9	100	26
	Haagen-Dazs vanilla ice cream, 4 fl. oz.	17.9	260	62
Eggs	Whole large egg	5.6	79	64
	Egg white (from 1 large egg)	0.0	16	0
Fats & Oils	Hellmann's Light reduced-calorie mayonnaise, 1 tbsp.	5.4	50	97
	Hellmann's Real mayonnaise, 1 tbsp.	11.3	100	100
	Crisco all-vegetable shortening, 1 tbsp.	11.9	110	97

Fats in Food (cont.)

Foods		Total fat in grams	Calories	% cal from fat
Fats & Oils (cont.)	Puritan 100% pure canola oil, 1 tbsp.	14	120	100
	Fleischmann's Diet reduced-calorie margarine, 1 tbsp.	6	50	100
	Land O Lakes margarine, 1 tbsp.	11	100	99
	Land O Lakes butter, 1 tbsp.	11	100	99
Snacks	Redenbacher's Original hot air-popped popcorn, 3 cups	0.7	68	9
	Redenbacher's butter-flavored microwave popcorn, 3 cups	6.6	132	45
	Bachman twist pretzels, 1 oz.	0.9	110	7
	Wise potato chips, 1 oz.	11.7	160	66
	Ritz crackers (four)	3.8	76	45
	Hershey's milk chocolate, 1 oz.	8.9	150	53
	Skippy creamy peanut butter, 2 tbsp.	16.8	190	80
Cookies & Cake	Oreo cookies (two)	4.4	106	37
	Sara Lee Original all-butter pound cake, 1 slice, 1 oz.	6.0	130	42
	Pepperidge Farm Milano cookies (two)	6.6	130	46

weight becomes harder and harder after a certain number of pounds have been shed—and why lost pounds almost inevitably return. The solution? Read on to see how exercise solves the problems caused by dieting and keeps lost pounds from coming back.

Exercise—The Vital Ingredient

Fortunately, the two problems created by dieting—a slower metabolic rate and the loss of calorie-burning muscle tissue—can be cured with a single solution: regular physical exercise.

If you truly want to lose weight and keep it off—permanently—you must make a long-term commitment to regular exercise in general and two types in particular: aerobic workouts and strength-training exercise. A single aerobic workout burns calories during the exercise session and for several hours afterward, and strength training helps preserve muscle that might otherwise be lost through dieting. *Combining* the two types of exercise can produce gratifying results, as the following study illustrates.

Researchers at the University of Massachusetts put thirty-eight obese, physically inactive women on a 1200-calorie-per-day diet and then divided them into four groups. Some of the women worked out aerobically on an exercise bicycle for half an hour three times a week, some of them spent the same amount of time doing strength-training exercises (weight lifting), other women split their thirty-minute exercise sessions into fifteen minutes of aerobics and fifteen minutes of strength-training exercise, and the rest of the women just dieted and did not exercise.

Five months later, the women who dieted but didn't exercise had lost about eight pounds, including a minimal amount of muscle mass. Almost all of the exercisers had lost more weight than the simple dieters had, and all of them had *gained* some muscle mass. The exercisers who had done both aerobic and strength-training exercise lost the most weight—an average of twelve pounds each.

Virtually all studies that have tried to find the secret to successful weight loss have come to the same conclusion: Many kinds of diet can help people lose weight. But to sustain that weight loss—to keep those pounds from sneaking back—you must combine dieting with exercise. The study described here shows that a particularly good exercise program may be one that combines aerobic exercises with a strength-training workout.

Emphasize Fiber

Perhaps the best way to ensure that you consume a low-fat diet is to eat more foods that are high in fiber. Foods that are rich in fiber—vegetables, fruits, grains, and beans—also tend to be low in both calories and fat. Switching from a typical American diet to one rich in these foods should definitely help you to lose more weight. Several clinical trials comparing similar weight-loss regimens have shown that adding fiber to people's diets helps them to lose an average of four additional pounds over a two- to three-month period.

Even if you don't lose weight on a diet rich in fiber, it will improve your health in other important ways. A substantial body of research shows that a high-fiber diet helps to reduce heart disease risk by lowering cholesterol levels, lowers the risk for diabetes, helps to prevent colon cancer, may help prevent breast cancer, and may reduce the risk for developing high blood pressure.

If you're like many people, your fiber intake is less than optimal. Half of all Americans consume less than 14 grams of fiber a day, while health experts typically recommend that healthy adults consume between 20 and 35 grams of fiber daily. To get more fiber, try complying with the U.S. Department of Agriculture's "Food Guide Pyramid," on the next page, which the agency published in 1992 to illustrate the government's idea of a nutritious diet.

The pyramid's foundation consists of six to eleven servings per day of grains—bread, cereal, rice, and pasta. All of these are potentially high in fiber if you choose whole-grain products. Stick with unrefined items such as whole-grain breads and whole-wheat pasta, brown rice, and cereals such as shredded wheat and bran flakes. You'll also get plentiful amounts of fiber from the pyramid's next level, consisting of three to five servings per day of vegetables and two to four servings of fruit.

If you've resolved to increase your fiber intake, don't go overboard. Consuming a lot more than the recommended maximum 35 grams of fiber daily can interfere with the body's absorption of calcium, iron, zinc, and other nutrients. And boost your fiber intake gradually, since doing it too fast can cause gas, bloating, cramping, or diarrhea.

It's More Than a Matter of Calories

So you've resolved to lose weight by adopting a high-fiber diet rich in whole grains, beans, fruits and vegetables, and low-fat dairy products. In that case, you're in for a bonus: This diet will not only help you shed pounds, thereby lightening the load on your

THE FOOD GROUP PYRAMID
A Guide to Daily Food Choices

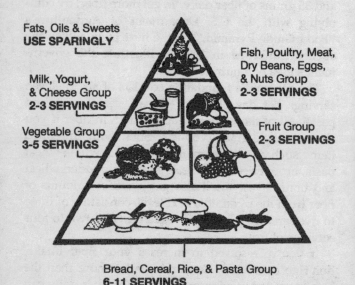

Fats, Oils & Sweets
USE SPARINGLY

Milk, Yogurt,
& Cheese Group
2-3 SERVINGS

Vegetable Group
3-5 SERVINGS

Fish, Poultry, Meat,
Dry Beans, Eggs,
& Nuts Group
2-3 SERVINGS

Fruit Group
2-3 SERVINGS

Bread, Cereal, Rice, & Pasta Group
6-11 SERVINGS

joints, but it offers nutrients that can keep osteoarthritis from worsening and may even help to prevent it. These nutrients for combating osteoarthritis are concentrated in four food groups: fruits, vegetables, dairy foods, and fish.

Eat More Fruits and Vegetables

A diet rich in fruits and vegetables provides you with antioxidants, the chemicals that can help to protect against not only osteoarthritis but a wide range of other chronic diseases associated with aging, including heart disease and several types of cancer. In particular, the antioxidants vitamin C and beta carotene are available in plentiful amounts from certain fruits and vegetables.

We need antioxidants to combat chemicals known as free radicals that are now suspected of playing a major role in causing these chronic diseases. As described in more detail in Chapter 5, the free radicals damage cell membranes, DNA, and proteins throughout the body. Recent research shows that diets high in antioxidants help protect people against the damage these free radicals cause, including the cartilage loss that occurs in osteoarthritis.

The antioxidants in food are the perfect complements to glucosamine and chondroitin sulfate, the dietary supplements that rebuild joint cartilage and that are the focus of this book. But many people don't eat enough fruits and vegetables to obtain the amounts of vitamin C and beta carotene they need.

The federal food pyramid calls for "Five a Day," or at least five servings daily of some combination of fruits and vegetables. But nutrition experts believe we should consume even more—at least seven servings of produce a day. Unfortunately, only one in five Americans eats five or more daily servings of fruits and vegetables, and a mere one in twenty of us consumes seven servings. The good news is that making fruits and vegetables a bigger part of your diet—and benefiting your joints and your overall health in the process—is not as hard as you may think. In fact, it can be surprisingly easy to fit in seven or more daily servings of fruits or vegetables, especially if you routinely eat three meals a day. You can begin boosting your fruit and vegetable intake right away by following these suggestions:

- Start your day with six ounces of one hundred percent fruit juice—just three-fourths of a cup—and you've taken care of one serving.
- Garnish your bowl of cereal with sliced bananas, berries, raisins, or other fruit. You only need a quarter cup of dried fruit, a half cup of berries, or one medium piece of a fruit such as a banana to make a full serving.
- Enrich your pancake or waffle batter with berries or sliced apples.
- Make your omelette with plenty of vegetables—onions, peppers, tomatoes, or any vegetable that appeals to you. Half a cup of chopped vegetables equals one serving. (To cut the fat and cholesterol in your omelette, make it with egg whites.)
- For lunch, make your salad out of chicory, romaine, or spinach. (Skip the iceberg lettuce, the least nutritious of all vegetable greens). One cup of raw leafy vegetables gives you one serving—which you can double by topping it off with just one-half cup of broccoli, carrots, celery, cucumber, mushrooms, peppers, or tomatoes.
- Adding a half cup of berries or a chopped piece of fruit to plain yogurt not only makes it tastier but provides you with a serving of fruit.
- You'll give color and texture to pasta salads by augmenting them with vegetables like broccoli, celery, and green and red peppers.
- Add tomatoes, sliced peppers, shredded carrots, or bean sprouts to sandwiches.
- When making pasta for dinner, remember that a half cup of tomato sauce qualifies as a serving of cooked vegetable.
- Add extra vegetables to stews, casseroles, and lasagna dishes.

- Make your soups thicker by adding finely chopped or pureed carrots.
- Begin most meals with a slice of melon, half of a grapefruit, or a half cup of fruit salad.
- Make cold fruit soups in the summer.
- Prepare several fruit desserts each week, such as poached pears or baked apples.
- If your dessert is frozen yogurt, add berries or sliced apples, bananas, peaches, or plums.
- When you're up for a healthy snack, don't just settle for sticks of celery or carrots. Enlarge your snack menu to include raw broccoli, cauliflower, green beans, summer squash, and red and green peppers.
- If you're brown-bagging your lunch, take along raw vegetables as a side dish.
- Rather than taking a coffee or tea break, drink fruit or vegetable juices. Stock up on small boxes or cans that are easy to carry with you.
- Take advantage of deli or supermarket salad bars when you don't have time to prepare a salad at home. (But avoid the items heavy with mayonnaise and dressings.)

You Can Do It

If you still doubt that seven servings of fruits or vegetables daily is feasible, consider this 1993 study involving forty volunteers who—like most of us—usually consumed less than four servings of produce a day. University of Minnesota researchers randomly assigned half the volunteers to receive instructions on boosting their intake to eight daily servings of fruits and vegetables, while the other twenty followed their usual diets.

After six weeks, the high-produce eaters had actually surpassed their goal. The food diaries they kept, as well as blood and urine tests, showed they were consuming on average more than nine servings a day, while produce consumption remained the same in the other group. The produce eaters reported no problems with either the cost or the added bulk of their new diets; most of them said they planned to continue eating at least six or seven servings a day after the study ended, and some even predicted they would have no trouble sticking with nine or more servings.

The Antioxidant Payoff from Produce

Once you eat fruits and vegetables, their antioxidants are released from the plant cells through digestion and are then absorbed into your bloodstream. From there they travel to the synovial lining of the joints and into the synovial fluid that bathes the cartilage—which is where they do battle with free radicals that are generated within the joints.

These free radicals contribute to osteoarthritis by damaging the proteoglycans and collagen, the key components of cartilage—but by consuming antioxidants, you can prevent the damage. A recent major study has shown that people who consume a diet high in antioxidants from fruits and vegetables have milder cases of osteoarthritis than people who don't take in many antioxidants. (See the discussion of the Framingham Heart Study in Chapter 5.) The study concluded that the major dietary antioxidants—vitamin C, vitamin E, and beta carotene—were all useful in protecting people against osteoarthritis.

Vitamin C. The Framingham research indicates that vitamin C is probably the key antioxidant for providing help against osteoarthritis. So it's definitely a good idea to consume lots of it in your diet. Fortunately that's not a difficult chore, since vitamin C is quite abundant in a nutritious, well-balanced diet. The table below lists examples of fruits and vegetables containing significant amounts of vitamin C.

If you comply with the latest dietary recommendations and eat five to nine servings of fruits and vegetables daily, you'll easily consume enough vitamin C to protect your joints. But if like many people you fall short on fruit and veggies, then you should consider taking vitamin C supplements, which are discussed in more detail in Chapter 5.

Beta Carotene. Until a few years ago, beta carotene supplements were all the rage, and vitamin-conscious people didn't think very much about getting this antioxidant from their food. Population studies had found that people whose diets were high in beta carotene were at low risk for developing several types of cancer, and bottles of beta carotene started flying off health food store shelves.

But as described in Chapter 5, recent clinical studies in which people were fed high doses of beta carotene in supplements found that beta carotene was not the panacea it was assumed to be—and that consuming a lot of it by taking supplements might actually be harmful. Of the three key antioxidants, beta carotene is the one you should try hardest to get enough of from your diet and not from tablets or capsules.

Found mainly in fruits and vegetables, beta carotene is part of the family of naturally occurring antioxidant substances called carotenoids. Beta carotene is the carotenoid most often studied, since it's the most plentiful of the carotenoids and the one most readily transformed into vitamin A.

According to current scientific thinking, beta carotene may not actually deserve the credit for the anticancer effects observed in studies that have measured people's dietary intake of beta carotene. Instead, those beneficial antioxidant effects may actually be due to the many other potentially nutritious substances—including other carotenoids—that are found in foods rich in beta carotene.

So while nutrition experts no longer recommend beta carotene supplements, they emphasize that it's still important to consume a diet high in beta carotene. They note that harmful effects from beta carotene have occurred only in studies where it's been used in *supplement form,* and that no studies have linked diets rich in beta carotene to any adverse effects whatsoever.

If you have osteoarthritis, try to capitalize on the antioxidant carotenoids by eating foods that are rich in beta carotene. While there is no official U.S. Recommended Dietary Allowance for beta carotene, nutrition experts suggest a daily dietary intake of about 5 to 6 milligrams. The table below shows that you should be able to meet that level pretty easily—sometimes with only a single item. Eating just one medium carrot, for example, gives you a beta carotene intake of 5.7 milligrams.

Vitamin E. Almost every month, it seems, a new study is published that finds yet another health benefit from consuming vitamin E. But while it definitely makes sense to include foods rich in vitamin E in your diet, that's not so easy to do. Some vegetables offer significant amounts of vitamin E, as shown in the table below. Unfortunately, however, the foods containing the most vitamin E are fatty foods such as nuts, seeds, avocados, and vegetable-oil products such as marga-

Vitamin C and Beta Carotene Content of Selected Fruits and Vegetables

PRODUCE WITH SIGNIFICANT AMOUNTS OF BOTH VITAMIN C & BETA CAROTENE

Food	Serving Size	Vitamin C (mg)	Beta Carotene[1] (mg)
Cantaloupe	1/2	75	4.8
Grapefruit, pink or red	1/2	47	1.6
Mango	1/2	29	1.4
Watermelon	1 slice	46	1.1
Bell peppers, sweet, red, raw	1/2 cup	95	1.1
Broccoli	1/2 cup	58	1.0
Sweet potato	1 medium	28	10.2
Kale	1/2 cup	27	3.0
Tomato juice	1 cup	45	2.2
Turnip greens	1/2 cup	20	3.9

PRODUCE WITH SIGNIFICANT AMOUNTS OF VITAMIN C

Food	Serving Size	Vitamin C (mg)	
Papaya	1/2	94	
Orange, California navel	1	80	
Kiwi	1	75	
Orange, Florida	1	68	
Strawberries	1/2 cup	41	
Brussels sprouts	1/2 cup	48	
Bell pepper, sweet, green, raw	1/2 cup	45	

**PRODUCE WITH SIGNIFICANT AMOUNTS OF
BETA CAROTENE**

Food	Serving Size		Beta Carotene (mg)
Apricots, dried	10 halves		6.2
Apricots	2		2.5
Carrot juice	1 cup		24.2
Chicory, raw	1 cup		6.2
Carrot, raw	1 medium		5.7
Spinach	½ cup		4.9
Pumpkin	½ cup		3.7
Collard greens	½ cup		3.4
Swiss chard	½ cup		3.2

[1]There is no official RDA for beta carotene, but the suggested daily intake for adults is 5 to 6 mg.

rine and salad dressing. But by choosing wisely, it is possible to increase your vitamin E intake while still keeping your fat intake low.

One recent study found that a typical low-fat, high-produce diet offers a daily intake of about 25 milligrams of vitamin E—approximately three times the Recommended Dietary Allowance. That's ample for avoiding a vitamin E deficiency, but it probably won't be enough to give you the benefit of vitamin E's potent antioxidant properties. For that you'll need a vitamin E supplement. Chapter 5 can help you choose a safe and useful vitamin E supplement dose, and the table below, which lists the vitamin E content of some selected foods, can help you choose foods that are low in fat but still contain significant amounts of vitamin E.

Vitamin E Content of Selected Foods

Food	Serving Size	Vitamin E (mg)	(IU[1])
Sunflower seeds	¼ cup	16	24
Filberts	¼ cup	8	12
Peanut butter	2 tbsp.	3	4
Wheat germ oil	1 tbsp.	26	39
Sunflower oil	1 tbsp.	7	10
Mayonnaise, regular	1 tbsp.	4	6
Margarine spread, light	1 tbsp.	3	5
Margarine spread, regular	1 tbsp.	2	3
Sweet potato, baked	1 medium	5	8
Avocado	1 medium	3	4

[1]Vitamin E content is often listed in International Units. (1 milligram of vitamin E equals approximately 1.5 IU.)
Source: ESHA Research, Salem, Oregon.

CAN OLESTRA WORSEN OSTEOARTHRITIS?

If you have osteoarthritis, you certainly don't want to be robbed of vitamins D and E. But olestra, the noncaloric artificial fat approved for use by the FDA in 1996, is being criticized for robbing the body of these and other important nutrients. Should you be concerned?

Since olestra is a fat, it's a magnet for fat-soluble vitamins—particularly A, D, E, and K—that it encounters in the intestinal tract. They're carried out of the body along with the olestra and therefore don't get absorbed into the bloodstream. If these vitamins and olestra are consumed at the same time, studies show, olestra can deplete their levels by up to thirty percent.

Procter & Gamble, the maker of olestra, has dealt with

that problem by fortifying the artificial fat with the very vitamins it tends to deplete. When olestra is saturated with these vitamins, it can't hijack the ones floating in the stomach.

To the critics of olestra, this "fix" is still inadequate. They say that Procter & Gamble has still done nothing about another class of nutrients that olestra depletes: the carotenoids. As noted earlier in this chapter, carotenoids (the best-known example is beta carotene) are compounds found in high amounts in green leafy vegetables and in fruit such as canteloupe and grapefruit.

Carotenoids may prevent certain types of cancers and help to minimize joint damage in osteoarthritis (see pages 95–96). At a 1996 press conference, professors at Harvard Medical School charged that widespread, long-term consumption of olestra might cause several thousand deaths yearly due to lung and prostate cancer and heart disease, plus hundreds of additional cases of blindness due to macular degeneration, an eye disease that primarily affects the elderly.

These claims seem overly alarmist. Olestra can "rob" your body of carotenoids only if it's swallowed at the same time they are. But if you eat your leafy salad more than an hour after your fat-free Pringles, the olestra should be long gone, no longer around to carry off carotenoids. And if you eat the recommended five servings of fruits and vegetables daily, you'll be consuming so many carotenoids that any losses to olestra will be trivial by comparison.

Favor Flavonoids, the Other Antioxidants

As a part of your effort to combat free radicals, you should also eat foods rich in flavonoids, antioxidant plant chemicals that are found in apples, celery, cranberries, grapes, and onions, as well as the beverages tea and red wine (red, not white wine, because flavonoids are concentrated in grape skins, which are not used in white wine). By attacking free radicals, flavonoids should not only help against osteoarthritis but will also provide protection against heart disease and cancer.

The strongest evidence for flavonoids' benefits comes from population studies of tea drinkers. Some studies show that regular tea drinkers have up to fifty percent less risk of developing certain cancers when compared with non-tea drinkers. It's believed that tea flavonoids help ward off cancer by preventing free radicals from damaging the DNA that controls cell growth. And a study of about eight hundred Dutch men found that the men who consumed the most flavonoids, mostly from black tea, reduced their risk of heart disease by two-thirds compared with men who consumed the least tea. The probable reason for the benefit: The "bad" LDL cholesterol that clogs arteries only does so after being chemically damaged by oxidation, and drinking green or black tea can prevent those destructive oxidative reactions.

Eat More Low-Fat Dairy Products

If you have osteoarthritis, you should certainly make sure that you're consuming the Recommended Dietary Allowance of vitamin D each day, which is 400 International Units. Judging by the results of the Framingham study on vitamin D and osteoarthritis (discussed in more detail in Chapter 5), that should provide enough vitamin D to keep your joints healthy.

You can readily obtain that amount of vitamin D by consuming a varied and nutritious diet that contains low-fat dairy products such as skim or one-percent-fat milk, yogurt, frozen yogurt, or cottage cheese. You can also get vitamin D from margarine and egg yolks. Vitamin D's importance in combatting osteoarthritis is discussed in more detail in Chapter 5.

Eat More Fish

Interest in the antiarthritic properties of fish stemmed from studies of Greenland Eskimos. Despite consuming a diet high in fat because they live mainly on fatty fish, the Eskimos were found to have a remarkably low incidence of heart disease. Further study showed that arthritis was also rare in these people. The beneficial effects from eating these cold-water fish were attributed to their oils—specifically the omega-3 fatty acids in fish oil.

Fish oil can help reduce inflammation, and several clinical studies have shown that fish oil supplements may offer modest benefits in easing the symptoms of arthritis. As described more fully in Chapter 5, most of these studies have involved patients with rheumatoid arthritis, so it's not clear whether people with osteoarthritis—which typically doesn't involve inflammation—will benefit from supplements.

Doctors who aren't convinced that fish oil supplements are a useful treatment for arthritis nevertheless encourage their patients to increase the amount of fish in their diet. They note that the Greenland Eskimos, whose high intakes of omega-3 fatty acids were associated with low rates of arthritis, are fish eaters and not supplement takers. All fish contain omega-3 fatty

Nutrient Value of Selected Seafood

Food (3 oz.)	Omega-3 fatty acids (gms)	Saturated fats (gms)	Total fat (gms)	Calories
Atlantic salmon	1.9	1.1	6.9	155
Herring	1.8	2.2	9.8	172
Whitefish	1.6	1.0	6.4	146
Bluefin tuna	1.3	1.4	5.3	156
Sardines, canned in oil	1.3	1.3	9.7	177
Mackerel	1.1	3.6	15.2	223
Sockeye salmon	1.1	1.6	9.3	184
Rainbow trout	1.0	1.4	5.0	128
Swordfish	0.9	1.2	4.4	132
Bluefish	0.8	1.0	4.6	135
Scallops	0.8	0.6	3.4	113
Bass, freshwater	0.8	0.9	4.0	124
Blue mussels, steamed (7)	0.7	0.7	3.8	146
Catfish	0.5	1.0	5.0	120
Halibut	0.5	0.4	2.5	119
Pollock	0.5	0.1	1.0	100
Sole/flounder	0.4	0.3	1.3	100
Ocean perch	0.4	0.3	1.8	103
Chinook salmon/lox, smoked	0.4	0.8	3.7	99
Alaskan king crab, steamed	0.4	0.1	1.3	82
Shrimp, steamed (15 med)	0.3	0.2	0.9	84
Clams, steamed (12 small)	0.2	0.2	1.7	126
Pacific cod	0.2	0.1	0.7	99
Tuna, canned in water	0.2	0.2	0.7	99
Haddock	0.2	0.1	0.8	95

acids to some degree, and fatty fishes such as bluefish offer the highest amounts.

The table below lists a number of fish and their amounts of omega-3 fatty acids, saturated fat, and total fat. Even if eating more fish doesn't help your arthritis, it does contribute to a healthy diet. A landmark study of American men found that those consuming the most fish were about forty percent less likely to die of a heart attack or a thrombotic (clot-caused) stroke over a six- to eight-year period than men who consumed the least fish. In addition, the omega-3 fatty acids in fish are now recognized as important nutrients for vision, for nerve and immune function, and for possible protection against several types of cancer.

Grab the Garlic

While the antioxidants are the most important dietary nutrients, they're not the only ones that can benefit people with osteoarthritis. The so-called allium vegetables—garlic, onions, chives, scallions, and leeks—may also be useful.

Allium vegetables are rich in sulfur compounds that are known to be beneficial for health. One of those compounds, allicin, reduces the liver's output of cholesterol—which explains why eating just half a clove of garlic per day can reduce cholesterol levels in the blood by about ten percent. But in addition, research suggests that these sulfur compounds may help to control arthritis symptoms, perhaps by correcting a nutritional deficit in people with arthritis.

Do Some Foods Cause Arthritis?

For many years, doctors treating patients with arthritis have dismissed the notion that diet has any effect on the disease. Nothing you eat can improve your condition, they've long insisted, and nothing in your diet can make your arthritis worse. But people who actually have arthritis have been just as adamant in claiming that diet can influence their disease, for better and for worse. And arthritis experts are finally acknowledging that the patients have been right all along.

For example, in a review article on dietary therapy for arthritis, published in 1991 in *Rheumatic Disease Clinics of North America*, the author concluded with this statement: "Although doctors understandably have been wary of the subject, sufficient orthodox studies now exist to suggest that diet may help at least a subgroup of patients."

Current thinking is that diet may affect arthritis in two major ways. On the negative side, some patients may be allergic to certain foods, and the symptoms they experience in their joints may be the result of their food allergies. There is also speculation that some foods, particularly members of the nightshade class of vegetables (see discussion below), may cause painful calcifications to occur in the joints. Alternatively, and on the positive side, certain foods such as fish oils may reduce inflammation.

So there are really two approaches to dietary therapy for arthritis: elimination therapy, in which potentially harmful foods are removed from the diet, and supplementation therapy, in which potentially beneficial foods are added.

Eliminate the Negative

Which of the many foods that you eat might be causing your aches and stiffness? There are basically two ways to find out. One is to eliminate the particular food from your diet that you suspect is the cause of your problems and then wait for a couple of weeks to see if you feel better. The more scientific way, known as dietary elimination therapy, should be done only under a doctor's supervision.

In dietary elimination therapy, you first eliminate from your diet virtually all foods that might be causing your symptoms. This can be as extreme as a total water fast lasting a week or a much more nourishing diet consisting of foods considered safe to eat, including fish, pears, carrots, and water. If your symptoms do disappear during that time, foods are then reintroduced one at a time to see which ones are actually causing the problem.

So far, the best evidence that reactions to foods can cause arthritis symptoms comes from studies involving people with rheumatoid arthritis, in which inflammation is largely responsible for causing damage to the joints. It's less clear whether allergies to foods play as great a role in osteoarthritis, where inflammation is usually less of a factor. But if you suspect that certain foods do cause your osteoarthritis to flare up, try eliminating them from your diet and see what happens.

In recent years, some people have claimed that when they eat vegetables that are members of the nightshade family—tomatoes, potatoes, eggplants, and peppers—their arthritis gets worse. Nightshade vegetables contain high levels of chemicals called alkaloids. These alkaloids could act to remove calcium from the bones and deposit it in the joints of certain people with arthritis, causing calcification, inflammation, and pain. Since these vegetables tend to be nutritious, you shouldn't convict—and evict—them from your diet without being quite confident that they're causing problems. But if you have some suspicions, it can't hurt to eliminate them for a couple of weeks and see if you feel better.

Chapter 8

Shake, Rattle, and Swim

If you have osteoarthritis, taking chondroitin sulfate and glucosamine can help restore lost or damaged cartilage and relieve your painful symptoms. But swallowing those nutrients won't help much unless they get absorbed by the cartilage in your joints—and that's where exercise comes in.

Pressure on the joint from exercise is vital in helping cartilage soak up chondroitin and glucosamine sulfate and other nutrients. But exercise is also important because it takes more than cartilage to make a healthy joint. Glucosamine and chondroitin sulfate may give you joints with the smoothest, strongest cartilage of anyone on your block. But if the muscles, tendons, and ligaments surrounding your joint are weak or inflexible, then pain and stiffness will still be your companions.

Finally, Exercise Is "In" for Arthritis

As joints become painful, we're tempted to avoid using them so as to ease the discomfort. But in doing so, we set ourselves up for a vicious cycle. Inactivity causes muscle wasting and weakness, which puts even more strain on the joints and causes more pain—making us even more disinclined to move our joints. Until very recently, doctors helped perpetuate this problem by advising their osteoarthritis patients to avoid exercise. Osteoarthritis, they assumed, was an inevitable result of aging, and exercise could only make things worse by speeding up cartilage destruction within the joints. But the advice to avoid exercise if you had osteoarthritis was very much off base. By now, research has shown that proper exercise not only won't hurt the joints, but can be absolutely vital in treating osteoarthritis. Consider the following benefits that exercise can offer:

- helps nourish cartilage and keep it healthy
- relieves pain
- improves flexibility
- strengthens muscles, tendons, and ligaments
- relieves the stress that can aggravate arthritis
- helps overweight people shed the extra pounds that may be the cause of their arthritis. (For people who are overweight and don't yet have arthritis, losing weight can help keep it from developing in the first place.)

And as a bonus, working out to help your osteoarthritis will enhance your overall health. Exercise can improve your immunity, lower your risk of developing heart disease, cancer, and diabetes, increase your overall fitness, relieve insomnia and depression, and improve your sense of well-being. (For further information on the psychological benefits that exercise can provide, see "Exercising your mind," below.)

When Stress Is Good

Whoever said "Use it or lose it" may have had the joints in mind. Unless you use your joints regularly, they'll lose their strength and resiliency and become weak, stiff, and ever more tender. Stretching exercises contribute by making the tissue surrounding the joint—its muscles, tendons, and ligaments—more flexible, which increases the joint's range of motion. But it's now clear that the joints must not only get in the habit of moving but must actually be stressed in order to become healthy and strong. Researchers refer to this stress on which the joints thrive as "repetitive joint loading."

The cartilage in our joints requires this repetitive loading to keep it structurally sound and to maintain the right mix of proteins, water, and other components of cartilage. For example, studies have shown that repetitive loading stimulates cartilage to produce more proteoglycans, one of the most important components of cartilage. (As described in Chapter 4, "The One-Two Supplement Punch," the nutritional supplements glucosamine and chondroitin sulfate are crucial building blocks for making proteoglycans.)

Research on animals has confirmed that keeping joints immobile can have a devastating effect on cartilage. When immobilized, cartilage produces fewer proteoglycans, and these all-important cartilage building blocks are soon in short supply, the water content of cartilage increases, and, ultimately, the cartilage softens and thins and erodes. Adding insult to injury, these changes make the cartilage much more vulnerable to injury if physical exertion is necessary—if a confirmed couch potato has to run for a bus, for example.

Keep in mind that cartilage is not solid like bone

but instead is supple and flexible, contracting and expanding like a sponge each time weight is applied to it. The cartilage in your knee, for example, compresses slightly each time you take a step, and then, as you step with your other foot, it expands to return to its resting shape. And since this spongy cartilage is bathed in synovial fluid, each step means that fluid is first soaked up by cartilage and then wrung out.

This repetitive soak/squeeze action not only helps lubricate the cartilage so that it doesn't dry out and become stiff, but it also feeds the cartilage. Unlike most other tissue in the body, cartilage isn't serviced by blood vessels that can supply the nutrients it needs but instead relies for its nourishment on nutrients in the synovial fluid. Only through joint loading that comes from weight-bearing exercise can cartilage maintain its health by soaking up those nutrients.

Weight-bearing exercise is simply any activity, such as walking or jogging, that makes your joints bear more weight than they would if you were sitting or standing still. Aerobic exercises and strengthening exercises, both of which are recommended for people with osteoarthritis, can give your joints all the jolting they need. One caveat: Be careful that the pounding your joints are subjected to is not too severe, or else you'll do more harm than good.

One other benefit of weight-bearing exercises also deserves mention: Such exercises also stimulate bone growth, which helps stave off the bone-thinning disorder osteoporosis.

Why You Must Stay Active

As people get older, they tend to lose the enthusiasm for physical activity that they had as children or young adults. But ironically, as you get older, staying active becomes more crucial than ever for maintaining good health. And that's especially true if you have osteoarthritis.

Researchers recently examined fifty adults with arthritis (all but four of them with osteoarthritis) for their susceptibility to heart disease. When compared with a group of nonarthritic people the same age, the people with arthritis were clearly worse off when it came to their risk factors for heart disease. They were much heavier, had higher blood pressures, higher blood-sugar levels (indicating possible diabetes), and lower levels of HDL cholesterol, the "good" form of cholesterol that helps prevent heart disease.

The explanation: People with arthritis tend to be inactive. "Risk factors for heart disease are affected by activity levels, and people who are active will be less likely to have abnormalities of the factors that promote heart disease," according to Dr. Edward Philbin, director of the heart failure clinic at the Mary Imogene Bassett Hospital in Cooperstown, New York, who conducted the study.

"It's been known for some years that osteoarthritis is associated with obesity, and obesity is related to cardiovascular disease," says Philbin. He puts part of the blame on doctors who often don't encourage their arthritis patients to exercise because movement causes them pain. But when people with arthritis do exercise, he says, they not only lower their risk of heart disease but can decrease their pain and improve their range of motion. "Studies have shown that when people with arthritis participate in exercise programs, they feel better, lose weight, and the symptoms of their disease often don't progress," he notes.

So if you've been letting your osteoarthritis keep

you on the sidelines, you've just run out of excuses for your inactivity. It's time to loosen up your joints and, by doing so, improve your heart's health and your overall health at the same time.

"Easy" Goes a Long Way

If you come away from this chapter with just a single message, we hope it's this: Exercise doesn't need to be strenuous to have a *major impact* on your osteoarthritis symptoms. This was clearly—even dramatically— illustrated in a study published in 1992 in the *Annals of Internal Medicine*. Researchers worked with 102 patients, forty to eighty-nine years old, who had been diagnosed with osteoarthritis in one or both knees. The patients were split into two groups. One group participated in an eight-week program of supervised fitness, walking three times a week, with each session no more strenuous than walking back and forth in a hospital corridor. People in the control group did not participate in the walking sessions.

After the eight weeks were up, people in the exercising group were functioning much better than at the start of the study. On average they had increased the distance they were able to walk in six minutes by nearly twenty percent. By comparison, people in the control group were able to cover less ground than they had eight weeks earlier. On an "arthritis pain scale," the walkers' pain had declined by twenty-seven percent. And the walking program provided these and other benefits without aggravating knee pain or triggering flare-ups.

A special message for couch potatoes: This study shows that you can keep your exercising to a walk and still help yourself. And for about the same amount of exertion, the stretching/strengthening exercises at the end of this chapter can ease the pain and increase the flexibility of joints from your neck down to your ankles. So don't get exercised about bringing some exercise into your life. The truth of the matter is that you can do a lot to help your joints without ever breaking a sweat.

Getting Started

If you're over forty, are planning to start a regular exercise program, and haven't had a checkup in more than two years—call and make an appointment before taking the plunge. A checkup is also advisable for anyone over forty who has one or more of the risk factors that increase their susceptibility to heart disease. You're at risk if you: smoke, are obese, have high blood pressure, diabetes, a family history of early heart attack, high levels of LDL or "bad" cholesterol, or low levels of HDL or "good" cholesterol. In addition, being physically inactive itself was recently classified as a risk factor for heart disease.

Depending on your present condition and your health history, your doctor may want you to take a stress test, to check on how your heart reacts when you exercise. To make certain you start in on the right foot, your doctor may refer you to a physical therapist, who can work with you to develop an exercise regimen suited to your particular joints.

Consulting a Physical Therapist

Physical therapists are exercise specialists who prescribe exercises to relieve pain and restore lost muscle and joint function. They can work with you to create a personalized regimen of stretching, strengthening, and aerobic exercises. Consulting a physical therapist can be especially helpful if your osteoarthritis is severe or if it's been a long time since you've done any exercise.

A course of physical therapy generally lasts just a few weeks, although long-term therapy may sometimes be advisable. Therapy sessions are scheduled anywhere from every day to once a week and typically last less than an hour. If you get a prescription from your doctor, the therapy is usually covered by Medicare and other insurance policies.

The physical therapists will give you a "fitness evaluation" that assesses several aspects of fitness including your aerobic capacity, sense of balance, the flexibility of all your joints, and your muscular strength. Then the therapist will work with you to develop a treatment plan targeted to the areas where you need help—walking or swimming to improve your aerobic capacity, for example, or flexibility exercises for a stiff knee. Ideally, the choices will include activities you enjoy, so that you'll be motivated to stick with the regimen for years to come. In addition to prescribing exercises, the therapist may also employ cold, heat, massage, ultrasound, or whirlpool baths to reduce pain and increase flexibility.

Your treatment plan should include well-defined goals and a timetable for improvements on your way to meeting those goals. If you're having trouble making progress, your therapist may be able to achieve better results by modifying your program. The ultimate aim of your course of physical therapy is to improve your physical condition to the point that you can exercise on your own.

The best way to find a physical therapist is to ask your doctor for a referral, and in some states a doctor's referral is required. All physical therapists must be licensed, and some are also certified by the American Board of Physical Therapy Specialists in fields including geriatrics, neurology, orthopedics, and sports. Physical therapists work in hospitals, clinics, health clubs, cardiac rehabilitation centers, nursing homes, and other settings. Some of them even make house calls.

Think Before You Exercise

Whether you consult a physical therapist or design your own exercise program, it's important to match your joints with the exercises that are most appropriate for them. If you have an arthritic shoulder, for example, you might benefit from stretching exercises but should avoid strenuous weight lifting. And if you have painful knees, participating in wind sprints is not a good idea. By showing common sense in the exercise you choose, you can help ensure that your workouts will improve your osteoarthritis and won't cause damage that could make things even worse.

Set Rational Goals

Once you start in, be sure to set reasonable goals for yourself. Being too ambitious—insisting you'll start off doing twenty push-ups or a hundred sit-ups, for example—almost guarantees that you'll abandon your workout program before you've given it a chance. You may well injure yourself from exertion you're not accustomed to, your aching body may resist taking another pounding, and you may well feel discouraged from having failed to meet your goals.

It's difficult at first to know how much exercise to do or when you have done too much. But here's a good rule for gauging whether you've overexerted yourself: If pain or discomfort from exercise lingers for more than two hours after your workout, then you have probably overdone things. While some muscle soreness is normal following unaccustomed exercise, you want to avoid a workout that causes pain, which is a signal that you're damaging your body. When it comes to exercising and osteoarthritis, "There's no gain without pain" should definitely NOT be your mantra.

Your strategy should be one of gradualism—to make each workout a little more strenuous than the next until you ultimately achieve your goal of "a good workout." For the first week or two, do your workouts at an easy pace and keep them brief, lasting no more than ten or twenty minutes. Then gradually extend the duration of your exercise sessions by no more than ten percent per week.

If you have been doing little exercise until now, you will reap tremendous benefit from a very modest program. Your first step should be to do the simple stretching and strengthening exercises on page 173 at least three times a week. Depending on your age and condition, these exercises might be supplemented with a daily walk. Only after a month on this regimen should you consider adding other, more strenuous forms of exercise to your program.

TIPS FOR EXERCISING SAFELY

As you embark on an exercise program, there is much that you can do to minimize the stresses you place on your joints. Here are some tips that can help:

- Protect your joints by being careful about the positions you get yourself into while exercising or doing chores or other activities. In particular, if you have osteoarthritis of the knee, avoid squatting, kneeling, and sitting in a cross-legged or yoga position.
- Wearing jogging shoes or other cushioned shoes when walking can soften the stress that footsteps put on your ankles, knees, hips, and spine.
- When you exercise, avoid high-impact exercises, such as sprinting or jumping rope, because they can damage arthritic joints.
- When your joint pain or discomfort is worse than usual, limit your exercises to stretching, then increase your activity level when your joints begin to feel better.
- If you're having a flare-up of joint pain, rest is certainly advisable. But avoid the temptation to rest your joints for long periods of time. Doing so can actually increase pain and stiffness. Remember that *not* exercising poses far more risk to osteoarthritic joints than does proper exercise.

Exercise and Weight Loss

One of the major attractions of exercise is its usefulness in helping you to lose weight. Being overweight is now regarded as a major cause of osteoarthritis. That's not surprising, since carrying around extra pounds puts significant strain on the joints—particularly the knees and, to a lesser extent, the hips. The good news: Losing weight is one of the best things that overweight people can do to treat their osteoarthritis. Weight loss can even prevent overweight people from developing the disease in the first place.

If you diet and don't exercise, your chances for sustained weight loss are practically nil. But if you exercise, you can lose a modest amount of weight even if you don't diet. Recently, researchers analyzed the combined results of twenty-eight clinical trials and found that men who worked out regularly for half a year lost an average of seven pounds. But if you want to lose more weight than that, you'll probably also have to go on a diet.

A combination of dieting and physical activity is clearly the best way to shed pounds and keep them off. And provided you work out consistently, even a moderate, low-intensity exercise program can reap big weight-loss dividends. For example, you can burn an extra thousand calories a week if you exercise thirty minutes a day doing such moderate activities as walking, gardening, yard work, or leisurely bicycling. Keep that up over the course of a year and you'll lose nearly fifteen pounds. And that means you've taken quite a load off of your joints.

Exercising Your Mind

Everyone feels down in the dumps some of the time. But for someone with a chronic health problem like osteoarthritis, feeling depressed or stressed or generally in a bad mood can get to be the norm. All the more reason, therefore, to get into the exercise habit. Recent studies show that exercise has a remarkable ability to smooth your moods—calming you down when you're stressed or tense and boosting your spirits when you're feeling depressed. It can also improve your self-confidence and even help you think better and be more creative.

Help for Anxiety. Exercise can reduce tension as effectively as traditional relaxation techniques such as meditation, according to a recent analysis of 159 studies on exercise's impact on anxiety. The emotional high from a single workout can last for several hours afterward, possibly much longer. Even more significantly, regular exercise has been found to curb anxiety even after the glow from a workout has faded, especially in people suffering from chronic anxiety. And programs that last longer than ten to fifteen weeks are more effective at reducing anxiety than are briefer programs.

Two types of exercise that help your osteoarthritis will also ease anxiety: continuous, rhythmic workouts like bicycling or swimming, and slow, meditative, stretching-type exercises such as yoga and tai chi. Although strength training appears to have little effect in reducing anxiety, mild to moderate activities like walking relieve anxiety at least as well as more demanding workouts.

Defeating Depression. Studies consistently show that people who are physically active are less depressed than inactive people. But is that because exercise actually reduces depression, or is it merely due to the fact that depressed people don't feel like exercising? To avoid that pitfall, ten studies have followed depressed volunteers as they either exercise, receive some other treatment, or just remain inactive. In all ten studies, exercise was found to significantly reduce mild to moderate depression. In addition, the three studies that compared exercise to psychotherapy found that exercise was at least as effective.

Any kind of exercise—strenuous or mild, rhythmic

or nonrhythmic—seems to lift depression. And it works not only for physically healthy people but also for people with arthritis and other chronic conditions.

In women, at least, regular exercise may even help prevent depression from developing in the first place. Researchers at the National Institute of Mental Health assessed the mood and habits of about 1,900 women and then reevaluated them eight years later. Among the women who weren't depressed at the start of the study, those who exercised at least occasionally were only half as likely to become depressed during the ensuing decade as those women who rarely or never exercised.

Improving Self-esteem. Even people who already feel pretty good emotionally can feel even better—have more confidence they can handle life's challenges—if they exercise. That's been shown by six clinical trials that tested the link between exercise and what's known as "self-efficacy." Similarly, other studies suggest that exercise raises self-esteem—especially when it comes to feelings about fitness and overall appearance.

If it does nothing else, a workout can provide an emotional lift. Even a brisk walk lasting ten minutes is enough to make you feel more relaxed and energetic, and regular workouts produce more lasting improvements. For example, researchers at the University of Washington assigned 121 older volunteers either to a lengthy program of walking and running or to a control group that didn't exercise. All participants were evaluated after one year, and the exercisers felt substantially better—less anxious, less lonely, more satisfied with life, and less worried about growing old—than the inactive group did.

Taking the Plunge

Three types of exercises—stretching, strengthening, and aerobic—should be included in a well-rounded exercise regimen.

Aerobic Exercises. Any exercise that raises your heart rate is an aerobic exercise, including walking. These exercises increase your overall fitness by training your heart and lungs to deliver oxygen more efficiently to the working muscles of the body. Aerobic exercises that involve weight bearing, such as walking or jogging, help to nourish and lubricate the all-important joint cartilage. In addition, aerobic exercises often serve as strengthening or stretching exercises for the joints. Swimming, for example, is both an excellent aerobic exercise and ideal for stretching. Walking and jogging are aerobic and also help build strength in leg and thigh muscles.

To improve your aerobic capacity, you should exercise at sixty to eighty percent of your maximum heart rate. This ideal range for aerobic exercising is called your target heart rate. (See box below, "Calculating your heart rate for aerobic exercise.")

Many different activities can give you a good aerobic workout, including bicycling, jumping rope, swimming, running, hiking, aerobic dancing, and cross-country skiing. But for people with osteoarthritis, walking and swimming are especially suitable. Walking is particularly good for people with osteoarthritis of the knees, who should avoid jarring activities. Water workouts, preferably in a heated pool, provide a great way for people with osteoarthritis to maintain or improve their mobility, strengthen their joints, and swim away from pain—all without putting undo strain on their joints, since the water helps to support their weight.

One rap against swimming has been that it doesn't provide as much aerobic training as working out on land. But a recent study at Temple University in Philadelphia has belied the standard wisdom and shown that water can offer a workout as aerobically effective as a vigorous workout on terra firma.

Researchers at Temple took a group of twenty older people and instructed ten of them to exercise in a pool three days a week and the other ten to remain inactive. The exercisers engaged in a spirited forty minutes of water aerobics that included kicking, twisting, hopping, and running in the water. Twelve weeks later, tests showed that the exercisers had improved their aerobic capacity—the ability of the heart and lungs to supply the muscles with oxygen—by fifteen percent, while there was no aerobic improvement in the control group. That gain is comparable to the improvement that older people can reap from a running program—but with far less stress on the joints.

CALCULATING YOUR HEART RATE FOR AEROBIC EXERCISE

To calculate your maximum heart rate, subtract your age from 220. For example, if you're forty-five years old, your maximum heart rate would be $220 - 45 = 175$ beats per minute. Then calculate the lower end of your target heart rate by taking sixty percent of 175, which equals 105. Calculate the upper limit of your target heart rate by taking eighty percent of 175, which equals 140. So, if you're forty-five, your target heart rate while exercising should be between 105 and 140 beats per minute. To improve your aerobic capacity, you should work out at your target heart rate for twenty to thirty minutes three times per week.

You can monitor your heart rate by finding your pulse, either by placing your fingertips on the palm side of your wrist or laying them lightly against the side of your voice box, counting the pulses for fifteen seconds, and then multiplying this number by four to get your pulse rate in beats per minute.

Stretching Exercises. These exercises move your joints through their full range of motion and, gently, even a bit further. And when you stretch a muscle slightly beyond its normal length, it gradually adapts to its new length. Numerous studies have shown that the muscle elasticity gained through stretching increases the range of motion of the joints. For people with stiffness due to osteoarthritis, doing stretching exercises offers an unsurpassed way to regain joint flexibility—which can make a world of difference in easing the most basic of tasks, from tying your shoelaces to scratching your back.

Stretching can bring other benefits as well:

- It can help protect you from injury caused by an abrupt or unaccustomed motion—reaching for a falling vase, for example, or slipping on the ice. If your muscles have been adequately stretched, they'll be less likely to suffer strains or tears when forced beyond their normal range of motion.
- When done before, after, and perhaps even while you're playing a sport or doing a strenuous workout, stretching can prevent what's technically known as "delayed-onset muscle soreness"—the aches and pains that turn up a day or two later.

- Regular stretching can help to ease everyday aches and pains caused by emotional stress or the stiffness from sitting in one place for too long.
- A good stretching routine is an excellent way to relax and to reduce stress—as exemplified by yoga, which both increases flexibility and enhances feelings of well-being.

To make sure your stretching program is successful, keep these four points in mind:

1. You can stretch in several ways, but the basic technique—called static stretching—involves gradually stretching through a muscle's full range of movement until you feel resistance or the first sign of discomfort. Hold this "maximum" position for ten to thirty seconds, relax, and then repeat this stretch several times.
2. To maintain the flexibility that you gain from stretching, you'll need to stretch at least three times a week.
3. After you've gotten the hang of stretching, try holding your maximum position for longer periods so as to increase flexibility even more. To gain significant increases in flexibility, you should hold stretches for one to two minutes.
4. Never bounce when you stretch—doing so can overstretch and injure muscles, tendons, or ligaments. Stretching should be done gradually and in a relaxed manner.

Strengthening Exercises. These exercises offer significant health benefits to people with osteoarthritis because they strengthen muscles, ligaments, and tendons—the tissues that support the joints. If you have osteoarthritis of the knee, for example, it clearly pays to strengthen your quadriceps muscle, the large muscle in front of your thigh. (It was the quadriceps tendon, which attaches the quadriceps muscle to the knee, that President Clinton tore in early 1997.)

To get an idea of what strength training can do for your osteoarthritis, consider the results of a study carried out recently at the State University of New York at Buffalo. Researchers put eighty people with osteoarthritis of the knee on a three-day-a-week strength-training program that involved weight lifting, isometric exercises, stationary bicycle riding, and endurance exercises. After three months on this strength-training regimen, ninety percent of the participants had less pain, eighty-five percent had improved the muscle strength around their knees, and ninety-five percent were better able to perform daily activities.

Strength-training exercises are crucial "antiaging" therapy. As we get older, we tend to lose muscle mass unless we participate in strength training. For people with osteoarthritis, strength-training exercises are especially important. They strengthen the muscles, tendons, and ligaments that move the joints and thereby increase mobility and decrease pain by taking stress off the bones in the joint.

The strength-training exercises recommended in this chapter focus on strengthening the all-important muscles and other tissues that surround the joints, and none of them requires any special apparatus. But your joints will be even better off if your muscle-strengthening efforts encompass your entire body. Why? Because increased overall strength can take some of the burden off your joints and protect them from injury.

Consider trying to open a living room window that's stuck shut. If you've strengthened your chest muscles, they can assume some of your lifting effort and reduce the stress and strain that would otherwise be placed on your elbows. That kind of strengthening program, known as weight training, usually requires equipment such as the barbells or Nautilus and other types of apparatus found in health clubs.

As with any other type of workout, it's best when beginning strength training to start in gradually. For each exercise—bicep curls, for example, or chest presses—choose a resistance level that permits you to do a set of eight to twelve repetitions. To keep building strength once you've reached twelve repetitions, you should increase the resistance again so you're back to being able to perform a set of only eight. For a further strength boost during your workout, once you've done your twelve repetitions, take off some resistance and then continue on for several more repetitions.

Be sure to work slowly to gain the full benefits of strength training. Try to make each repetition last about six seconds—two seconds for the first half of the maneuver and another four seconds for the return to the original position.

How often and how intensely should you do strength training? That depends on your particular goals. Even a single session per week will help to slow muscle loss and may stop it entirely. And working out twice per week provides nearly as much benefit— three-fourths as much muscle building—as a three-times-per-week schedule. As for intensity, studies indicate that one set of each exercise appears to be just as effective as several sets, at least for the first few months. After that, it's not clear whether multiple sets provide any advantage. Unless you feel the need to keep building more and more muscle, a single set of each strength-training exercise during your workout should probably be ample.

Know When to Rest

As important as exercise is, there are times when the best thing you can do for your joints is to rest them completely. Anyone with osteoarthritis learns that some days are better than others—and for no apparent reason. In learning how to manage with osteoarthritis, one of the most difficult lessons is figuring out how to strike a balance between overdoing it on the one hand and retreating from life on the other.

Rest, of course, is very important—and like most everyone else, people with osteoarthritis get too little of it. Shooting for seven or eight hours of sleep a night is a good goal, but a large majority of Americans fail to get that much. Sometimes it's best, if you can manage it, to set aside several rest periods in your daily schedule. A short nap during the day can also work wonders on your physical as well as mental condition.

There may be occasions when you don't need to rest your entire body, but feel distressed by a particular joint. In that case, some form of splinting might be in order. You may have an image of splinting as something you learned about years ago in first-aid class, involving a thin piece of wood and adhesive tape, but today's splints are much more sophisticated.

Splints work their pain-relief magic by keeping a painful or stiff joint out of action for a while. They're typically used on the hands and wrists by people with arthritis, particularly those who have rheumatoid arthritis. If you think your osteoarthritis could benefit from judicious splinting, ask your doctor to refer you to a physical therapist, who can measure and fit you for the right device and show you how to use it.

Exercises That Stretch and Strengthen

When it comes to exercises for your joints, some of them do double duty—simultaneously stretching the joint to increase flexibility and strengthening the muscles, tendons, and ligaments that bend the joint. Most of the ones described below fall into that two-for-one category. These exercises are among the ones that physical therapists recommend for people with osteoarthritis.

Except where noted, you should do these exercises twice a day, morning and night. Start in gradually, at first doing only two or three repetitions of each exercise; then slowly increase your number of repetitions until, for each exercise, you're obtaining the maximum benefit by doing three sets of ten repetitions (thirty repetitions in all) per exercise session. (For the hip rolls, just one set of ten rolls daily should be sufficient to relieve stiffness.)

To strengthen your joints further, do the exercises with weights strapped on your legs; alternatively, try working against the resistance offered by an elastic band. You can buy weights as well as elastic bands in most sporting-goods stores.

Knee Exercises

Quad tighteners. Lie on your back, prop yourself up with your forearms, and then extend one leg. Bend your other leg to protect your back. Tighten the thigh muscle of your extended leg; note that this action should push the back of your knee down to the floor.

Then switch legs and repeat to complete one repetition.

Foot lifts. Place a firm pillow under one knee and lie flat on your back. Bend the other leg. Without moving your knee off the pillow, slowly raise your foot until your leg is straight.

Extend and flex. Sit in a chair and, keeping your feet flat on the floor and your thighs on the chair, straighten one leg so that it's parallel to the floor. Hold that position for three to five seconds, then bend your knee and slowly return your foot to the floor. Then repeat with the other leg.

Reach for the stars. Lie on your back with one knee bent and the other extended as straight as possible on the floor. Now bend the knee of the straight leg, bringing it as far toward your chest as you can. Next, straighten that leg, pushing out with your heel, so that your foot points directly upward. Finally, lower the leg to the floor. Repeat again with the same leg but this time pushing your leg out at a different angle. Repeat three to five times, extending your leg at a different angle each time. Then do the same routine with the other leg.

Quad builder. Lie on your back with one leg bent. Flex back the foot of your other leg (i.e., point your toes back toward your head), tighten your knee so the leg is straight, then lift that leg until your foot is two feet off the floor. Count slowly to five, then lower the leg slowly, touching the floor with your calf first. Repeat with your other leg.

Hip Exercises

Side leg lifts. With your head propped up with one hand, lie on your side with the leg you want to exercise on top. (Bend your lower leg slightly to maintain balance.) Being careful to keep your top leg straight and without moving it forward, lift it about two feet off the floor and then slowly lower it. Repeat with the other leg.

Hip rolls. Lie on your back and extend both legs. Rotate one leg inward, then rotate it outward. Repeat with other leg.

Thigh lifts. Sit in a chair with both of your feet flat on the floor. Raise the knee of your affected leg as high as possible, then slowly lower it.

Hip flex. Lie on your stomach on the floor or bed. Keeping your knee straight, lift one leg just a few inches off the ground, count to ten as you hold that position, and then slowly let your leg return to the floor. Repeat with the other leg.

Neck Exercises

Stare down. Looking straight ahead with your chin slightly dropped, bend your head forward, keeping your chin tucked in. Then straighten your head *but don't bend it backward*.

Look both ways. Begin by looking straight ahead, with chin dropped slightly. Turn your head and look over your left shoulder, then turn it so you're looking over your right shoulder.

Tick tock. Begin by looking straight ahead with your chin slightly dropped. As you continue looking straight ahead, bend your head sideways so that your ear moves toward your shoulder. (Don't lift your shoulder toward your ear.) Then bend your head to the other side.

Shoulders and Elbows

Shoulder touch. Sit or stand with your arms at your sides, palms facing backward. Lift both arms forward to shoulder level with palms facing down. Now turn your palms up, and touch your fingertips to your shoulders, allowing your elbows to drop. Straighten both arms at shoulder level, turning your palms down. Lower your arms slowly, first to your side and behind your back, and then touch your palms together.

Shoulder circle. Make sure your shoulders are relaxed as you look straight ahead. Then roll both shoulders in circular movements—forward, up, backward, and down.

Touch down! Sit on a stool or other hard surface with your back straight, your feet flat on the floor, and your hands on your knees. Then touch your stomach, keeping your elbows out to the side. With elbows still out to the side, touch your shoulders, then touch behind your head. Finally, stretch both arms upward with your palms facing each other, then lower your arms back to your knees.

Back

Pelvic tilt. Lie on your back with your knees bent and feet flat on the floor. Press your back against the floor as you tighten your stomach. Hold this position for a count of ten, then relax.

Body curl. As you flatten your back against the floor in the pelvic tilt position described above, slowly bring your knees toward your chest, using your hand to pull your knees even closer to your chest. Hold this position for a count of ten, your knees slightly separated as you do so. Then slowly allow your feet to return to the floor.

Leg slides. Starting in pelvic tilt position, slowly slide one foot away from you until your leg is straightened, then slowly pull it back to the bent knee position, keeping your back pressed to the floor the entire time. Repeat with the other foot.

Curl and slide. Lie on your back with your knees bent. Bring one knee toward your chest and hold it with both hands. Then, with your back pressed to the floor, slowly slide your other foot along the floor until that leg is straight; with your back still pressed against the floor, slowly slide that leg back until it returns to the knee-bent position. Then switch legs and repeat.

The Buddha. Sitting with your legs crossed in front of you, hold your feet with your hands. Slowly lean forward, moving your face toward the floor. Don't jerk or bob.

Chair bend. Sit with your feet flat and your hands on your hips. As you look straight ahead, bend your trunk to one side. Then straighten and bend over to the other side.

Run Hot and Cold Against Joint Pain

Whether your joints are sore from doing exercise or just plain sore, heat or cold or a combination of the two can help to soothe the discomfort.

Heat. Applying heat—taking a hot bath or applying a heating pad, for example—is a great way to relax stiff muscles and soothe aching joints by stimulating blood circulation in the area. But warmth penetrates less than half an inch below the skin surface. It won't touch deeper joints such as the hips or knees, but it can reach joints closer to the surface, particularly the knuckles and other joints of the hand. That's why people with osteoarthritis of the hands may find relief with heated mittens or by immersing their hands in warm water.

A somewhat messier alternative is to dip your hands into warm paraffin. With a paraffin bath, you dip your hand or other affected joint into a small vat of melted wax mixed with mineral oil, remove it from the bath, and then peel off the material after its heat is no longer warming the joint. Your doctor can give you instructions on how to make a paraffin bath at home.

Some people may find relief from a deep-heat treatment called diathermy, in which devices produce heat of different wavelengths including shortwave, microwave, or ultrasound. But these treatments can be expensive (they're usually available only in doctors' offices or clinics), and may not be worth the cost. In two clinical studies, some people with osteoarthritis of the knee did exercises to strengthen the muscles around their knees, while others took diathermy treatments before doing the knee exercises. Neither study found that diathermy relieved pain any more effectively than the exercises alone.

Cold. When a joint is acutely painful or inflamed, cold treatment is a better treatment than heat. Cold relieves pain by reducing inflammation and swelling and raising the pain threshold by numbing the nerves that sense pain. It's also a good treatment for relieving muscle aches after strenuous exercise. A quick way to make an ice pack is to fill a small sealable plastic bag with ice. Or if ice isn't handy, you can improvise by wrapping a bag of frozen vegetables in a towel and applying this "veggie pack" to your painful joints.

You may also find that alternating cold and heat treatments provides better relief than does using either of them alone. For example, you can apply a heating pad for fifteen minutes, let your joint rest for five minutes, and then apply an ice pack for another fifteen minutes.

If you do use cold or heat, take some precautions. Apply cold or heat for only fifteen to twenty minutes at a time, and be sure that a towel or other barrier comes between your skin and the cold or heat source. Any form of heat has the potential for causing burns. Anyone whose sensation is impaired, such as people who have diabetes, should be especially careful about possible overheating.

Chapter 9

Nontraditional Arthritis Therapies

Back in 1984, the U.S. Congress's House Subcommittee on Health and Long-term Care issued a lengthy report entitled "Quackery: A $10 Billion Scandal." The subcommittee estimated that older Americans spent that amount each year on worthless pills, devices, and other remedies—with much of that money being spent on useless treatments for arthritis.

From the standpoint of con artists, arthritis is a near-perfect ailment, with desperate people seeking relief from a disease that has no cure. As a result, many doctors who treat patients with arthritis lash out in almost knee-jerk fashion against any new therapy that doesn't have immense amounts of clinical data in support of it. But with their blanket condemnations of all things new or different, doctors may not always be serving the best interests of their patients.

It's certainly true that many unconventional treatments for arthritis don't work, and some can actually be harmful. That's why doctors have long warned their patients not to trust anything that hasn't been exhaustively tested in controlled clinical trials and approved for use by the Food and Drug Administration. But by insisting that unproven is the same as ineffective, doctors have reflexively pooh-poohed some therapies that are turning out to be quite useful—better and safer, in fact, than the drugs that doctors have traditionally relied on.

So it has been heartening—and surprising—to observe the medical community's reaction to glucosamine and chondroitin sulfate, the dietary supplements that are revolutionizing osteoarthritis treatment and are the focus of this book. These products will never gain the endorsement of the FDA as "safe and effective" since, as dietary supplements, the FDA doesn't regulate them that way. Yet several osteoarthritis experts in this country have said they are so impressed with results in patients who are taking the supplements that they're now studying the supplements in clinical trials—and some have begun taking them for their own osteoarthritis.

Even the conservative Arthritis Foundation—which essentially defines arthritis quackery as everything not yet etched into medical textbooks—has been surprisingly upbeat in its reaction to glucosamine and chondroitin sulfate. The foundation has acknowledged that glucosamine has "the potential to slow the degradation of cartilage" and has "anti-inflammatory properties" as well. As for the clinical studies conducted on glucosamine and chondroitin sulfate over the past fifteen years, the foundation has acknowledged that they "show some promise"—high praise indeed from this organization.

In this chapter we'll tell you about some other ways of treating osteoarthritis that are also promising although not yet in the mainstream of therapy. We'll describe other treatments that have helped some people but that you may want to think carefully about before trying. And since hype is inevitably mixed with hope when it comes to osteoarthritis, we'll also warn you about some treatments that promise much more than they can deliver.

Opt for Acupuncture?

If you have osteoarthritis that hasn't responded to traditional therapies, you may want to consider getting treatment from a qualified acupuncturist.

Acupuncture is the branch of Chinese medicine in which needles are inserted into the skin to treat various disorders or to relieve pain. The treatment is based on the notion that the Chi, or life force, flows through the body along meridians, or channels. Ill health results from blockage in one or more of these meridians, and it's possible to restore health by inserting needles at appropriate sites on the affected meridians and successfully unblocking the meridians. These sites are known as acupuncture points.

Western medicine has taken a skeptical view of acupuncture ever since it gained popularity in the U.S. in the 1970s, and many doctors continue to question its use. Nevertheless, research on acupuncture indicates how the therapy might actually work: It causes the central nervous system to release morphinelike substances called endorphins, which act as natural painkillers.

Acupuncture has been successfully used as an anesthetic for dental procedures and in surgical operations as well as during labor and delivery. It's also used to relieve chronically painful conditions such as arthritis that don't respond to standard treatments. And a well-designed study presented at the 1996 meeting of the American College of Rheumatology indicated that acupuncture can indeed provide significant pain relief for people with osteoarthritis.

The study, conducted at the University of Maryland School of Medicine, involved seventy-four patients whose knee osteoarthritis caused them moderate to severe pain despite their use of NSAIDs. The patients were split into two groups: One continued treatment with their NSAIDs; the other group took NSAIDs along with traditional Chinese acupuncture administered twice a week for eight weeks by a licensed acupuncturist. By the end of the study, the patients receiving NSAIDs plus acupuncture were experiencing significantly less pain as well as improved flexibility and walking ability. By contrast, the patients treated only with NSAIDs had gotten no better.

Recently acupuncture took a big step toward greater acceptance by the medical community. In 1996, the FDA lifted the "investigational use" designation from acupuncture needles and reclassified them as "general use" medical devices. Supporters of acupuncture hope that this policy change will put pressure on insurance companies to cover acupuncture treatments.

Acupressure. Acupressure is very similar to acupuncture but without the needles. Instead, the hands and fingers are used to apply pressure at acupressure points on the body. Of course, acupressure does enjoy one advantage over acupuncture: You don't need to go to a practitioner for acupressure but can instead perform it on yourself—either on the genuine acupressure points or directly on your joints.

Whether you use an acupressurist or perform the

therapy on yourself, acupressure is similar to various forms of massage in that it uses different rhythms, pressures, and techniques. When the joints aren't tender, you may prefer vigorous, firm pressure applied to a particular spot for three to five seconds. A more gentle technique uses a firm, gentle touch for a minute or more. Although we're not aware of any studies involving acupressure and osteoarthritis, the recent success of acupuncture in treating osteoarthritis suggests that acupressure might hold promise as well.

For help in locating the acupressure points, you should consult a book on acupressure. A particularly good one is *Arthritis Relief At Your Fingertips: Your Guide to Easing Aches and Pains Without Drugs,* by Michael Reed Gach in cooperation with the Acupressure Institute of America (Warner Books, paperback, $15.99).

The Usefulness of Yoga

It's no stretch to say that yoga is proving effective at relieving the pain of osteoarthritis. The word yoga means "union," and the practice of this Hindu discipline is aimed at uniting the mind and the body. Whether or not you embrace the mystical side of yoga, many of the postures or positions it employs are tailor-made for alleviating the symptoms of osteoarthritis.

Some of these yoga positions are virtually identical to the range-of-motion exercises that physical therapists recommend. Others help to strengthen the muscles, tendons, and ligaments that surround the joints. And almost all of them help to reduce stress and create a feeling of relaxation.

The exercises performed in yoga are done *slowly*, and while you're doing them you focus on breathing deeply and evenly. There is no bouncing, no jerky movement, no straining to perform a certain number of repetitions or achieve some goal within a certain amount of time.

If you do take up yoga, be aware that certain positions may not be appropriate for your particular joint problems and could actually aggravate them. If you have osteoarthritis of the knee, for example, you should probably avoid the lotus, or sitting, position, since it may put undue strain on your knee joints. To be on the safe side, it may be best to get expert guidance on positions from a yoga instructor, preferably one who has experience working with arthritis patients.

In a recent nationwide survey of people with arthritis, eighty-eight percent who had tried yoga reported that they had obtained temporary or lasting relief from it. And in a study involving people with osteoarthritis of the fingers, researchers at the University of Pennsylvania School of Medicine found that patients who took the yoga training could move their fingers more easily and experienced less pain and tenderness than patients treated only with drugs. The researchers concluded that yoga is a "potentially valuable new approach" to managing osteoarthritis.

For best results with yoga, you should practice it regularly—for up to an hour a day, if possible. But if you can't spare that much time, doing shorter, daily sessions lasting fifteen minutes or so is probably more useful than scheduling longer sessions only a couple of times a week.

It makes perfect physiological sense that yoga can

ease the symptoms of osteoarthritis. Just as a hot bath can soothe pain by relaxing tight muscles in the joints, a relaxation technique like yoga helps to lower stress all over the body by relieving muscle tension and reducing the heart rate and blood pressure.

There are many different relaxation techniques besides yoga, but all of them involve breathing slowly and deeply and thinking peaceful thoughts. You don't need any fancy facilities to practice relaxation. A quiet spot anywhere will do—in your home, outdoors, or even in your car.

Chiropractic

Manipulation, particularly of the spine, is a widely accepted therapy. The health profession that puts the most emphasis on manipulation is chiropractic, from the Greek, meaning "done by hand."

So far, manipulation has proven useful against the one malady you'd most expect it to help: back pain. A study issued in 1991 by the prestigious Rand Corporation concluded that manipulation is appropriate for patients with common, acute low-back pain that has been present for three weeks or less.

What about chronic pain experienced by people with osteoarthritis? A recent clinical trial concluded that patients with chronic back and neck pain showed greater improvement with manipulation than with conventional physical therapy or conservative medical treatment. And now it's turning out that the real value of manipulation for osteoarthritis might not be in pain relief but rather in relieving stiffness: In clinical studies, high-tech force detectors have shown that the chiropractic thrust—a small, quick maneuver, lasting but a fraction of a second, which moves the joint past its normal range of motion—improves the mobility of the joints of the spine.

Keep in mind that chiropractors aren't the only health care professionals who offer manipulation. Some orthopedic surgeons, osteopaths, and physical therapists also use manipulation to relieve pain and restore joint function.

Take the Waters?

Spas—thermal spring waters—have long been used to treat many diseases. Just how useful spas are for treating osteoarthritis has been unclear, and some experts have derided spa therapy for osteoarthritis as merely an expensive form of relaxation. But in early 1997, the *British Journal of Rheumatology* published the first study on whether spas help in treating osteoarthritis. The joint-warming therapy produced some heartwarming results.

The study involved 188 French patients with osteoarthritis of the knee, spine, or hip who were divided into two groups. One group spent twenty-one days at the famous spa resort of Vichy, France, where they experienced various types of hydrotherapy including underwater massage and hot mud packs. The other group—the control group—maintained their normal routines of daily living. All patients were evaluated before the study and again three weeks and six months afterward. People in the control group didn't become measurably better or worse over that time; by comparison, the spa attendees were in less pain, had more mobility, needed lower doses of pain-relieving drugs, and generally had a better quality of life. In addition, these benefits were prolonged—still measurable six months after the people had been at the spa.

To Tens or Not to Tens

Transcutaneous electrical nerve stimulation, more commonly known as TENS, is a controversial method for relieving the severe and persistent pain of osteoarthritis and other health problems. It involves applying minute electrical impulses to nerve endings lying beneath the skin. A TENS unit—a battery-operated device about the size of a pack of cigarettes—transmits these electrical impulses to electrodes that are placed on the skin or sometimes surgically implanted in the body.

Several studies have looked at the usefulness of TENS for treating osteoarthritis. The best-designed of these studies involved fifty-six patients who had suffered for at least six months with symptoms caused by osteoarthritis of the knee or hip. After being assigned to use either a TENS unit or a sham unit that didn't emit any impulses, they took the devices home and were asked to use it for thirty minutes twice daily. After using the devices for six weeks, seventy-four percent of patients using a TENS unit reported more than a twenty-five percent reduction in pain, while only twenty-eight percent of patients using the sham device reported that much improvement.

Overall, studies indicate that TENS proves helpful for about sixty percent of people using it for pain relief. For some the relief is temporary, lasting only as long as the treatment does; for others, the pain relief persists for a while after treatment. One caution: TENS should never be used by someone with a cardiac pacemaker, since the electrical impulses from the unit could interfere with the pacemaker's function.

Homeopathy

Over the past few years, homeopathic remedies have become extremely popular, available not only in health food stores but displayed in the aisles of many pharmacies as well. These products are promoted for healing a wide variety of ailments, including arthritis. A couple of years ago, in an issue of *Let's Live* magazine, a leading homeopath estimated that there are 150 homeopathic remedies being sold for different types of arthritis.

Homeopathic remedies are based on a medical system developed in the late 1700s by a German physician, Samuel Hahnemann. He was horrified at the harsh treatments used in his day, in which patients were bled or dosed with toxic purgatives and poisons, and he worked to devise a gentler form of medicine.

Hahnemann said that a substance, such as coffee, that caused a symptom, such as agitation, when given in large amounts, could cure the same symptom when given in negligibly small amounts. Today, his proponents liken the main tenet of homeopathy, "like cures like," to immunology, which creates immunity in people through injection of small amounts of a disease-causing microbe.

But the homeopathic dosage is minuscule compared with what is in a vaccine. And, in fact, homeopaths contend that the less concentrated the dose, the more potent the medication. That explains why some homeopathic remedies are diluted to the point that in some cases not a single molecule of the active substance remains.

Even homeopathy's leading advocates admit that they don't know how homeopathy works, but they point to a number of recent studies—involving asthma, diarrhea in children, and other ailments—in which homeopathic remedies performed significantly better than placebos. We're not aware of any studies that have looked at homeopathic remedies for use in treating osteoarthritis or any other form of arthritis. But regardless of their effectiveness, homeopathic remedies are extremely safe and therefore shouldn't make anyone's arthritis worse.

Copper Bracelets

The ancient Greeks wore copper bracelets to relieve aches and pains, and the notion that copper can help against arthritis has persisted through the centuries. The most that can be said for copper bracelets is that some are attractive and none will hurt you. But, unfortunately, there is no evidence that copper bracelets help against osteoarthritis and no physiological reason why they should.

DMSO

DMSO is an industrial solvent similar to turpentine. In the 1960s, DMSO was touted as a possible treatment for a number of health problems, including arthritis. But a panel of experts appointed by the National Academy of Sciences concluded that DMSO is both useless and potentially dangerous in the treatment of arthritis.

The solvent, which can act as a local anesthetic and is readily absorbed through the skin, has received FDA approval as a drug for treating a single health problem: a rare bladder disease called interstitial cystitis. Some veterinarians use DMSO to treat bruises in dogs and horses, but humans should stay away from the stuff.

Bee Venom

It's a sign of how debilitating arthritis can be that some people purposely try to get stung by bees in their quest for pain relief. Even more distressing is the fact that the benefits that some people claim to derive from bee stings may require several thousand stings over the course of a year.

Not only is the evidence for a benefit from bee stings practically nonexistent, but anyone who gets stung by a bee risks an allergic reaction that can include anaphylactic shock, which can be fatal. We recommend against using bees for your knees—or any other joint, for that matter.

Honey and Vinegar

Credit for this strange concoction probably belongs to Dr. D. C. Jarvis, whose 1960 book, *Arthritis and Folk Medicine*, introduced the world to folk remedies that Vermonters had relied on for two hundred years for the treatment of arthritis. Believers contend that the vinegar thins the body fluids, allowing stiff, painful joints to move more freely. The recipe—two teaspoons of honey and two teaspoons of apple-cider vinegar dissolved in a glass of water—is easy to follow, but actual benefits are as rare as palm trees in the state's capital of Montpelier.

Chapter 10

Promises for the Future

All of the standard treatments for osteoarthritis do little more than minimize the symptoms. The hope for the future lies in new therapies that get at the underlying cause of osteoarthritis: the breakdown of the cartilage that covers the ends of bones in the joints.

As we have noted in this book, the dietary supplements glucosamine and chondroitin sulfate do exactly that. They help to halt the breakdown of cartilage and actually stimulate the growth of new cartilage. The great advantage of these two supplements is that they're both found naturally in human cartilage and appear quite safe to use, even in high doses.

In addition to rebuilding their cartilage the natural way, people with osteoarthritis may soon be able to choose from among several high-tech "cartilage repair" methods that are now being investigated. These and other innovative and experimental treatments for osteoarthritis are discussed below.

Autologous Chondrocyte Transplantation. Some 200,000 people a year with cartilage problems such as osteoarthritis may be able to benefit from a still-experimental technique called autologous chondrocyte transplantation, in which cartilage grown in the laboratory is transplanted directly into the joint where it's needed. The technique, developed by Swedish doctors, begins with removal of a sample of a patient's healthy cartilage. That sample is then "grown" in a laboratory, and when enough new cartilage cells, known as chondrocytes, are available, the cartilage tissue is inserted into the joint where it's needed. Since the implanted cartilage tissue is autologous—that is, the patient's own—there is no risk that the immune system will reject it.

So far, the technique has been used mainly on people with damaged knee cartilage. Doctors trained in the procedure remove a tiny chunk of cartilage, containing several thousand cells, from the patient's knee, and then send it to a laboratory where the cartilage cells are cultured in a petri dish. The cells multiply, increasing by about a thousandfold, until more than 100 million of them are present. At that point, the laboratory freezes the cells and mails them back to the patient's doctor. Then comes the reinsertion, in which the doctor surgically opens the joint, stitches or otherwise packs the new cartilage in place, sews the knee back up, and then puts it in a brace to stabilize it while the new cartilage takes hold.

The total cartilage replacement procedure can cost up to $50,000, and since doctors have only been doing it for about five years, it's not yet known how durable the new cartilage will be. Keep in mind that the technique has proven most useful in repairing injuries involving small, localized cartilage defects; it's unclear how effective it will prove to be for correcting the more generalized cartilage breakdown that's involved in osteoarthritis. But the technique does seem promising, and some orthopedic surgeons in the U.S. have started using it on patients with osteoarthritis.

Donor Cartilage. In another technique aimed at replacing damaged or destroyed cartilage, researchers at Jefferson Medical College in Philadelphia have successfully replaced bone and cartilage cells in a mouse by giving it cells removed from a donor mouse. Regarding the possible use of this technique in people, the researchers have said it would probably first be tried on children with genetic diseases that have caused them to be born with defective bone or cartilage. In an effort to cure their disease, these children would receive cartilage cells from normal human donors.

Ultimately, the donor cartilage procedure may be used to replace lost or damaged cells in people whose osteoarthritis has a genetic basis. And it may even be possible to carry out the procedure using one's own cartilage cells, following gene therapy to correct the genetic defect responsible for the disease. These "corrected" stem cells would then be transplanted back into the person's body, where hopefully they would begin to produce normal cartilage cells.

Replenish the Fluid. Treat osteoarthritis pain with an injection? That's the principle behind Synvisc, a viscous and elastic fluid that is injected into osteoarthritic knees to supplement the synovial fluid that surrounds the joints. Synvisc is enriched with a synthetic variant of hyaluronic acid, which is found naturally in synovial fluid but that tends to degrade in joints afflicted with osteoarthritis.

Treatment consists of three injections spaced one week apart. Clinical studies that have so far involved about 1,000 patients have shown that Synvisc relieves pain and allows for freer knee movement. In the future, Synvisc may be tested in other joints, including the hip and ankle.

So far, Synvisc has been approved for use in Canada, Sweden, and the People's Republic of China, and approval in this country might not be far off. In November 1996, an advisory panel to the Food and Drug Administration recommended that the agency approve Synvisc for use in the U.S. The agency is not bound by recommendations from its advisory panels, but usually concurs with them.

Growth Factor Paste. A "paste" spiced with a substance that promotes the growth of cartilage cells has successfully healed cartilage injuries and prompted growth of new cartilage in laboratory animals. The substance is a growth factor called transforming growth factor beta (TGFB) that is found naturally in the body.

The paste formed new cartilage in the animals and healed defects in their cartilage, and these cartilage improvements were still present when the animals were examined a year later. Further studies must be done in both animals and people to assure that this growth factor paste is safe, effective, and practical. But if the paste proves out, it could help restore the cartilage in people with osteoarthritis.

TGFB is also the focus of research by a team of doctors in the U.S. and Switzerland. But rather than mix it into a paste, these researchers packaged TGFB into liposomes—tiny bubbles with synthetic membranes—and injected the liposomes into the damaged cartilage of animals. The liposomes acted like timed-release capsules, slowly releasing their TGFB "payloads" and stimulating cartilage repair.

Low-Intensity Pulses. Electromagnetic fields are usually regarded as things to be avoided—especially the ones created by overhead power lines or household appliances. But recent research suggests that pulsed electromagnetic fields could be quite useful for treating osteoarthritis patients.

In one study, a team led by Johns Hopkins University researchers studied whether low-intensity electromagnetic fields could help patients with osteoarthritis of the knee. Forty-one patients underwent treatment with a portable, battery-powered device that was worn over their knee and emitted a low-intensity electromagnetic field. Another thirty-seven patients—the control group—wore identical devices that were inactive. For four weeks, patients in both groups wore the devices for six to ten hours a day, with most patients actually sleeping with the devices attached.

The patients were evaluated weekly during the study and again six months after the study ended. In the evaluation, a physician assessed the severity of the patients' osteoarthritis and the patients themselves rated their pain and how well they could function. All three measures—the physician's assessment and the patients' rating of their pain and mobility—reflected improvement to some degree in the group treated with the electromagnetic fields. Patients using the device for more than six hours per session experienced the most improvement.

Researchers aren't sure how electromagnetic fields help against osteoarthritis, but they suspect that the fields may stimulate cartilage cells to produce more cartilage. Regardless of the mechanism involved, pulsed electromagnetic fields do seem to help patients with osteoarthritis. They are as effective as drugs in relieving osteoarthritis symptoms—and probably much safer, since the pulsed fields are not known to cause any adverse side effects.

Gene Therapy. In 1990, a study in the *New England Journal of Medicine* showed that osteoarthritis can be caused by an inherited genetic abnormality. It confirmed what had long been suspected—that some cases of osteoarthritis are genetic in nature. The gene defect was found in a family whose members developed osteoarthritis at an early age, due to abnormally soft cartilage.

The problem was traced to a mutation within a gene that forms type II collagen, a crucial component of joint cartilage. More recently, researchers have found several other genes that, when mutated, may cause osteoarthritis. At least one-fourth of all cases of osteoarthritis may be found to have a genetic basis, experts say, raising the possibility of curing them through gene therapy.

Gene therapy uses sophisticated techniques to "correct" mutations within genes. By correcting the mutation, gene therapy may result in a cure by allowing the gene to produce a normal protein rather than the abnormal one responsible for the disease. Already, several laboratories are working on gene therapy for osteoarthritis.

At St. Jude's Hospital in Memphis, Tennessee, researchers have begun a clinical study of gene therapy that could lead to gene therapy for people with osteoarthritis. The study involves children with osteogenesis imperfecta, the result of a genetic defect that produces fragile bones that fracture easily.

The first children enrolled in the study are being treated with donated "normal" cells, but there's a risk that the recipient's immune system will reject the donated cells as foreign. The goal is to rely entirely on a patient's own cells: removing them, repairing the genetic defect, and then putting the cells back into the patient. If these trials go well, this gene therapy method could be applied to osteoarthritis patients in as little as two years.

New Drugs

Better NSAIDs. Nonsteroidal anti-inflammatory drugs (NSAIDs) continue to be a mainstay of arthritis treatment. NSAIDs work by inhibiting production of hormonelike chemicals called prostaglandins, which play major roles in causing pain and inflammation.

But unfortunately, as we've seen, NSAIDs don't discriminate between the prostaglandins they affect. They also shut down "good" prostaglandins responsible for the mucus that protects the stomach lining from the corrosive effect of stomach acid—which explains why gastrointestinal irritation often accompanies treatment with NSAIDs. Now, several pharmaceutical companies are working to develop a new type of NSAID that would be more selective, inhibiting only the prostaglandins involved in pain and inflammation and leaving other prostaglandins unaffected. (The use of NSAIDs for treating osteoarthritis is discussed in more detail in Chapter 3.)

Cytokine Blockers. Much of the damage in osteoarthritis probably results from destructive enzymes that are released either by the cartilage cells or by the synovium, the tissue that lines the joint. Such tissue breakdown is actually a necessary function—part of a dynamic breakdown/buildup process that allows tissues and organs to continually regenerate themselves.

The destructive action of these enzymes (including protease, which breaks down protein, and collagenase, which breaks down collagen) is normally balanced by cartilage production. But cartilage destruction—osteoarthritis—can result when these enzymes destroy cartilage faster than it can be rebuilt.

One way that glucosamine and chondroitin sulfate work to restore cartilage is by blocking these enzymes, and alternative ways of doing the same thing are now being investigated. One strategy is to block the chemicals, known as cytokines, that trigger production of the destructive enzymes. The treatment approaches involve gene therapy and new drugs.

Researchers are using gene therapy to inactivate a key enzyme-triggering cytokine known as interleukin. In this work, so far limited to animals, the researchers first remove cells from the animals' synovium—the cells suspected of releasing enzymes that break down cartilage. These cells are then "supplemented" with a gene that makes a protein that inhibits interleukin's production. Finally, the cells are put back into the joint and rejoin the synovial lining. The hope is that cells deprived of the ability to make interleukin can no longer pump out cartilage-destroying enzymes, either.

Several drugs have shown promise in blocking these cytokines or actually wiping out the cartilage-destroying enzymes themselves. One of them, now being investigated in both test tube and animal studies, is the antibiotic tetracycline. Other drugs that may help include a class of drugs called heparinoids and two experimental NSAIDs, tiaprofenic acid and tenidap.

Someday there will be a cure for osteoarthritis, thanks to these therapies or others not yet envisioned.

In the meantime, you can take advantage of the most promising solution currently available: the dietary supplements glucosamine and chondroitin sulfate. Clinical studies have shown not only that both supplements are safe but that they can ease the symptoms of arthritis by actually helping to rebuild cartilage.

You can continue to be informed about the latest developments in osteoarthritis research and treatment by contacting the information resources listed in the following section.

Resources

General Arthritis Resources

The Arthritis Foundation
1314 Spring Street
Atlanta, GA 30357-0667
Tel: 800-283-7800

This national nonprofit organization sponsors research on arthritis, educates the public about the disease, and sponsors continuing education for professionals. The Foundation offers informational material and support to patients through a number of venues: patient support groups, lectures, and abundant literature, including self-help materials and a series of patient brochures on numerous topics related to arthritis. Many local chapters sponsor activities such as swimming and self-help classes. For information, contact one of the Foundation's local offices, write or call the Foundation's headquarters in Atlanta, or browse the foundation's excellent web site.

Arthritis Society of Canada
National Office
250 Blair Street East
Suite 901
Toronto, Ontario M4W3P2
Tel: 416-967-1414

Sponsors public education programs as well as continuing education for professionals, raises money for research, and publishes patient information materials.

National Arthritis and Musculoskeletal and Skin Diseases Information Clearinghouse
National Institutes of Health
1 AMS Circle
Bethesda, MD 20892-3675
Tel: 301-495-4484
Sponsored by the National Institute of Arthritis and Musculoskeletal and Skin Diseases, a part of the National Institutes of Health. Offers an annotated bibliography of materials on osteoarthritis and other arthritic conditions as well as useful information packages, including "Arthritis in General" and "Arthritis and Diet."

American College of Rheumatology
60 Executive Park South, Suite 150
Atlanta, GA 30329
Tel: 404-633-3777
The professional organization of rheumatologists, dedicated to treating and studying all forms of arthritis. Can provide a list of rheumatologists by state.

Support Groups

When people with a health problem need advice or reassurance, they may turn to family members or a physician. But in addition, many people are helped by sharing their experiences and concerns with others who have the same problem, as part of a support group.

Over the past decade, the number of support groups has increased tremendously, and there are now groups devoted to virtually every health problem, including arthritis. Support groups provide therapy in the form of mutual support: people talking, listening, asking questions of each other, and, above all, providing the kind of encouragement that's only possible among people with intimate knowledge of a particular health problem.

Support groups are especially useful for the help they can offer in solving problems. At arthritis support group meetings, these may include practical problems such as the best way to deal with morning stiffness or interpersonal issues such as how to talk to a spouse about sharing household chores with you.

For information on finding a support group in your area, contact your local chapter or the national headquarters of the Arthritis Foundation (see above) or:

The National Self-Help Clearing House
25 West 43rd Street
New York, NY 10036
Tel: 212-354-8525

Pain Clinics

Many people with osteoarthritis have chronic pain that can't be relieved with drugs. They may be helped considerably by one of the more than one hundred accredited pain clinics around the country. These clinics employ therapies as varied as biofeedback and surgery and most are staffed by professionals from a number of disciplines—neurologists, psychiatrists, psychologists, physical therapists, and others. They can help wean patients from bad habits (narcotic addiction, for example) and teach techniques for controlling pain. In addition, most pain clinics sponsor patient self-help groups.

For information on finding an accredited chronic pain management program in your area, contact:

The Commission on Accreditation of Rehabilitation Facilities
4891 E. Grant Road
Tucson, AZ 85715
Tel: 520-325-1044

Other Organizations

The American Chiropractic Association
1701 Clarendon Boulevard
Arlington, VA 22209
Tel: 800-986-INFO
Information on chiropractic and how to find a chiropractor in your area.

The American Physical Therapy Association
1111 North Fairfax Street
Alexandria, VA 22314
Tel: 703-684-APTA
Information on finding a physical therapist in your area, plus information about physical therapy, including the organization's free pamphlet, "Fitness: A Way of Life."

The Foundation for Human Understanding
P.O. Box 1009
Grants Pass, OR 97526
Tel: 541-597-4360
Information on meditation.

The Integral Yoga Institute
227 West 13th Street
New York, NY 10011
Tel: 212-929-0586
Information on yoga.

The National Council Against Health Fraud
P.O. Box 1276
Loma Linda, CA 92354-1276
Tel: 909-824-4690
Information about questionable treatments for arthritis or other health problems.

The organizations listed below can send you useful information on massage therapy:

American Massage Therapy Association
820 Davis Street, Suite 100
Evanston, IL 60201
Tel: 708-864-0123

American Oriental Bodywork Therapy Association
Glendale Executive Campus
1000 White Horse Road
Vorhees, NY 08043
Tel: 609-782-1616

Associated Bodywork and Massage Professionals
28677 Buffalo Park Road
Evergreen, CO 80439-7347
Tel: 303-674-8478

Using the Internet

Having a computer and a modem allows you to go online for a wealth of information about osteoarthritis and other health problems. A convenient way to access it all is by subscribing to one of the major online service providers such as America Online (AOL), Compuserve, or Prodigy.

AOL's Personal Empowerment Network (Keyword PEN) is a particularly impressive resource. Once you're there, you'll see a list of health-related topics including "Arthritis and Related Concerns." Click on that and you'll be presented with a pull-down menu offering additional information on arthritis such as "Arthritis-Related Articles" and "Muscle- and Joint-Related Articles" plus links to arthritis-related sites on the World Wide Web, including "Knee Replacement," "Hip Replacement," and "Rheumatoid Resources."

AOL's Personal Empowerment Network also lets you search the massive MEDLINE database for studies on arthritis or any other health topic, access software libraries that offer thousands of easy-to-download health-related resources that can run on Macintoshes or PCs, and enter chat rooms where people discuss a wide variety of health topics.

Another advantage to being online is that you can tap into any one of several thousand newsgroups. People congregate in newsgroups to chat about a variety of topics related to a central theme, such as arthritis. The newsgroups truly are forums for the free exchange of ideas, opinions, and questions. Whatever topic you're interested in, there's sure to be a newsgroup that covers it. Of the hundreds of newsgroups accessible through AOL and other online services, the one called "alt.support.arthritis" may be the most useful for people with osteoarthritis.

There you can read message "threads"—discussions that typically begin with someone asking a question, which in turn stimulates responses from others who are participating in the newsgroup. On a recent visit to the alt.support.arthritis newsgroup, we saw interesting message threads on dozens of issues including "NSAID-induced stomach ulcers," "dealing with pain," and the search for "affordable glucosamine."

Another useful feature of AOL and the other online services: They give you access to the rest of the Internet, including sites on the World Wide Web. There are literally thousands of web sites, but some that are particularly relevant to people with osteoarthritis include the following:

The Arthritis Foundation
http://www.arthritis.org
This is probably the best web site for people interested in any form of arthritis, including osteoarthritis. From this site you can download (i.e., transfer from the web site to your computer) copious amounts of information—new research findings, practical advice, fact sheets, statistical information as well as position papers that the Arthritis Foundation has issued on various treatments.

Health Web's Rheumatology Page
http://www.medlib.iupui.edu/hw/rheuma/
home.html
This site is a collaborative effort between the Ruth Lilly
Medical Library and the Health Web project.

Want to read what the Merck Manual has to say
about osteoarthritis? Interested in the American College of Rheumatology's recent treatment guidelines
and position statements? They're both in "Rheumatic
Disease Resources," one of several useful offerings on
the Rheumatology Page, including: "Electronic Publications" (arthritis-related journals and newsletters
available on the Internet), "Electronic Communica-
tions" (information about electronic discussion
groups and newsgroups), and "Miscellaneous Resources" (patient support groups, drug databases, and
other related resources).

Health World Online
http://www.healthy.net
This site, which calls itself the "Home of Self-Managed
Care," looks at osteoarthritis and other disorders
mainly from a holistic standpoint. It includes a health
food store in cyberspace from which you can order a
wide variety of supplements, including seven different
glucosamine products, with just a few keystrokes.

**Doctor's Guide to the Internet/Arthritis
Information & Resources**
http://www.pslgroup.com/arthritis.htm
This site offers you medical news and alerts, arthritis
information, drug information, and information about
newsgroups and other arthritis-related web sites.

Shape Up, America!
http://www.shapeup.org/sua/
Shape Up, America! was founded by former surgeon general C. Everett Koop to encourage Americans to eat less, exercise more, and lose weight. As one of its most useful offerings, this site calculates your Body Mass Index (BMI) for you. All you have to do is enter your height and weight. BMI, a ratio between a person's height and weight, is a better indicator than weight alone for predicting a person's risk for osteoarthritis, heart disease, adult-onset diabetes, and other diseases associated with being overweight. After it has calculated your BMI for you, this web site tells you your level of risk, ranging from "minimal" to "extremely high."

References

Chapter 1.
"Arthritis: The Chronic-Care Challenge of the 21st Century." Media briefing sponsored by the American Medical Association, New York City, Nov. 16, 1995.

"Arthritis prevalence and activity limitations—United States, 1990." *Journal of the American Medical Association*, vol. 272, no. 5, 1994.

Brandt, Kenneth D. "Nonsurgical management of osteoarthritis, with an emphasis on nonpharmacologic measures." *Archives of Family Medicine*, vol. 4, Dec. 1995.

Cartilage Degeneration in Osteoarthritis: Unravelling the Mystery. Basle, Switzerland: Ciba-Geigy Limited, 1988.

Clayman, Charles B., ed. *Bones, Muscles, and Joints*. Pleasantville, NY: Reader's Digest, 1992.

Felson, David T. "The epidemiology of osteoarthritis: Prevalence and risk factors." In *Osteoarthritic Disorders*, ed. Klaus E. Kuettner and Victor M. Goldberg. Rosemont, IL: American Academy of Orthopaedic Surgeons, 1995.

Felson, David T., et al. "Weight loss reduces the risk for symptomatic knee osteoarthritis in women." *Annals of Internal Medicine*, vol. 116, no. 7, 1992.

Hochberg, Marc C., et al. "Guidelines for the medical management of osteoarthritis. Part I. Osteoarthritis of the hip. Part II. Osteoarthritis of the knee." *Arthritis & Rheumatism*, vol. 38, Nov. 1995.

Koopman, William J. "Rheumatology." *Journal of the American Medical Association*, vol. 265, no. 23, 1991.

"Targeting the debilitating effects of arthritis." Posting on Arthritis Foundation web site, quoting statistics from the U.S. Centers for Disease Control and Prevention, 1996.

Chapter 2.
"Arthritis in General." National Institute of Arthritis and Musculoskeletal and Skin Diseases, National Institutes of Health, Nov. 1996.

Clayman, Charles B., ed. *Bones, Muscles, and Joints*. Pleasantville, NY: Reader's Digest, 1992.

Dieppe, Paul. "The classification and diagnosis of osteoarthritis." In *Osteoarthritic Disorders*, ed. Klaus E. Kuettner and Victor M. Goldberg. Rosemont, IL: American Academy of Orthopaedic Surgeons, 1995.

Gregg, Daphna W. "Arthritis: A Harvard Health Letter Special Report." Boston: Harvard Medical School Health Publications Group, 1995.

Kantrowitz, Fred G. *Taking Control of Arthritis*. New York: HarperCollins, 1990.

Knowlton, R.G., et al. "Genetic linkage of a polymorphism in the type II procollagen gene (COL2A1) to primary osteoarthritis associated with mild chondrodysplasia." *New England Journal of Medicine*, vol. 322, 1990.

"Reporter's Guide to Arthritis and Other Diseases of the Joints, Muscles & Bones." The American College of Rheumatology, 1994.

Chapter 3.
Bradley, John D., et al. "Comparison of an antiinflammatory dose of ibuprofen, an analgesic dose of ibuprofen, and acetaminophen in the treatment of patients with osteoarthritis of the knee." *New England Journal of Medicine*, vol. 325, 1991.

Clough, John D., et al. "The new thinking on osteoarthritis." *Patient Care*, Sep. 15, 1996.

"Drugs for rheumatoid arthritis." *The Medical Letter on Drugs and Therapeutics*, vol. 36, Nov. 11, 1994.

Fennerty, M. Brian. "Nonsteroidal anti-inflammatory drugs, ulcers and histamine-2 blockers." *Archives of Internal Medicine*, vol. 153, Nov. 8, 1993.

Griffin, Marie R., et al. "Practical management of osteoarthritis: Integration of pharmacologic and nonpharmacologic measures." *Archives of Family Medicine*, vol. 4, Dec. 1995.

Griffin, Marie R. "Nonsteroidal anti-inflammatory drug use and increased risk for peptic ulcer disease in elderly persons." *Annals of Internal Medicine*, vol. 114, no. 4, 1991.

Oliwenstein, Lori. "Spell relief with over-the-counter pain pills." *American Health*, Jan./Feb. 1996.

Skolnick, Andrew A. "Rheumatologists issue guidelines for preventing and treating corticosteroid-induced osteoporosis." *Journal of the American Medical Association*, vol. 277, no. 2, 1997.

Wilcox, C.M., et al. "Striking prevalence of over-the-counter nonsteroidal anti-inflammatory drug use in patients with upper gastrointestinal hemorrhage." *Archives of Internal Medicine*, vol. 154, 1994.

Chapter 4.
Cartilage Degeneration in Osteoarthritis: Unravelling the Mystery. Basle, Switzerland: Ciba-Geigy Limited, 1988.

Caterson, Bruce and Clare E. Hughes. "Anabolic and catabolic markers of proteoglycan metabolism in arthritis." In *Osteoarthritic Disorders*. Rosemont, IL: American Academy of Orthopaedic Surgeons, 1995.

Conte, A., et al. "Biochemical and pharmacokinetic aspects of oral treatment with chondroitin sulfate." *Arzneim.-Forsch./Drug Res.*, vol. 45 (II), no. 8, 1995.

Crolle, G. and E. D'Este. "Glucosamine sulphate for the management of arthrosis: a controlled clinical investigation." *Current Medical Research and Opinion*, vol. 7, no. 2, 1980.

Drovanti, A., et al. "Therapeutic activity of oral glucosamine sulfate in osteoarthritis: A placebo-controlled double-blind investigation." *Clinical Therapeutics*, vol. 3, no. 4, 1980.

Fioravanti, A., et al. "Clinical efficacy and tolerance of galactosaminoglucuronoglycan sulfate in the treatment of osteoarthritis." *Drugs Exptl. Clin. Res.*, vol. 17, no. 1, 1991.

Gross, D. "*Orale chondroitinsulfatemedikation zur behandlung von arthrosen*." *Therapiewoche*, vol. 33, no. 33, 1983.

Hanson, R. Reid. "Oral glycosaminoglycans in treatment of degenerative disease in horses." *Equine Practice*, vol. 18, Nov./Dec. 1996.

Mazieres, B., et al. *"Le chondroitine sulfate dans le traitement de la gonarthrose et de la coxarthrose."* *Revue du Rhumatisme*, vol. 59, July–Sept. 1992.

Muller-Fassbender, et al. "Glucosamine sulfate compared to ibuprofen in osteoarthritis of the knee." *Osteoarthritis and Cartilage*, vol. 2, 1994.

Pipitone, V.R. "Chondroprotection with chondroitin sulfate." *Drugs Exptl. Clin. Res.*, vol. 17, no. 1, 1991.

Plaas, Anna H.K. and John D. Sandy. "Proteoglycan anabolism and catabolism in articular cartilage." In *Osteoarthritic Disorders.* Rosemont, IL: American Academy of Orthopaedic Surgeons, 1995.

Pujalte, Jose M., et al. "Double-blind clinical evaluation of oral glucosamine sulphate in the basic treatment of osteoarthritis." *Current Medical Research and Opinion*, vol. 7, no. 2, 1980.

Soldani, G. and J. Romagnoli. "Experimental and clinical pharmacology of glycosaminoglycans (GAGs)." *Drugs Exptl. Clin. Res.*, vol. 17, no. 1, 1991.

Tapadinhas, Macario Joao, et al. "Oral glucosamine sulphate in the management of arthrosis: report on a multi-centre open investigation in Portugal." *Pharmatherapeutica*, vol. 3, no. 3, 1982.

Vaz, Antonio Lopes. "Double-blind clinical evaluation of the relative efficacy of ibuprofen and glucosamine sulphate in the management of osteoarthritis of the knee in out-patients." *Current Medical Research and Opinion*, vol. 8, no. 3, 1982.

Chapter 5.
"Alzheimer's progression may be eased by vitamin E." *New York Times*, Apr. 24, 1997.

"Antioxidants—Sorting out the A, B, C's—and E's." *News Snacks*. Robert W. Woodruff Health Sciences Center, Nov. 1994.

Kolasa, Kathryn M., et al. "When patients ask about vitamin-mineral supplements." *Patient Care*, Sept. 15, 1996.

McAlindon, Timothy E., et al. "Relation of dietary intake and serum levels of vitamin D to progression of osteoarthritis of the knee among participants in the Framingham Study." *Annals of Internal Medicine*, vol. 125, no. 5, 1996.

―――. "Do antioxidant micronutrients protect against the development and progression of knee osteoarthritis?" *Arthritis & Rheumatism*, vol. 39, no. 4, 1996.

Recommended Dietary Allowances, 10th ed. Food and Nutrition Board, Commission on Life Sciences, National Research Council. Washington, D.C.: National Academy Press, 1989.

Chapter 6.
Beren, J.J., et al. "Therapeutic effect of Cosamin on autoimmune type II collagen-induced arthritis in rats (abstract)." Presented at the North American Veterinary Conference, Jan. 11–15, 1997.

Brody, Jane E. "Taking an alternative path to search for relief for arthritic knees. *New York Times*, Jan. 15, 1997.

Bucci, Luke. *Nutrition Applied to Injury Rehabilitation and Sports Medicine*. Boca Raton, FL: CRC Press, 1995. (See Chapter 12, "Glycosaminoglycans.")

Foreman, Judy. "People, and their pets, tout arthritis remedy." *Boston Globe*, Apr. 9, 1997.

Karzel, K. and R. Domenjoz. "Effects of hexosamine derivatives and uronic acid derivatives on glycosaminoglycane metabolism of fibroblast cultures." *Pharmacology*, vol. 5, 1971.

Setnikar, I., et al. "Pharmacokinetics of glucosamine in man." *Arzneim-Forsch./Drug Res.*, vol. 43 (II), no. 10, 1993.

Chapter 7.
"American College of Rheumatology Position Statement: Diet and Arthritis." *Rheumatic Disease Clinics of North America*, vol. 17, no. 2, 1991.

Darlington, L. Gail. "Dietary therapy for arthritis." *Rheumatic Disease Clinics of North America*, vol. 17, no. 2, 1991.

Darlington, L.G. and N.W. Ramsey. "Review of dietary therapy for rheumatoid arthritis." *British Journal of Rheumatology*, vol. 32, no. 6, 1993.

Guthrie, Helen A. *Introductory Nutrition*, 7th ed. St. Louis: Times Mirror/Mosby College Publishing, 1989.

McCarthy, Geraldine M. and Dermot Kenny. "Dietary fish oil and rheumatic diseases." *Seminars in Arthritis and Rheumatism*, vol. 21, no. 6, 1992.

Panush, Richard S. "Does food cause or cure arthritis?" *Rheumatic Disease Clinics of North America*, vol. 17, no. 2, 1991.

Whitney, Eleanor N., et al. *Understanding Nutrition*, 5th ed. New York: West, 1990.

Chapter 8.
"Arthritis and Exercise." National Institute of Arthritis and Musculoskeletal and Skin Diseases, National Institutes of Health, Feb. 1997.

Brandt, Kenneth D. "Nonsurgical management of osteoarthritis, with an emphasis on nonpharmacologic measures." *Archives of Family Medicine*, vol. 4, Dec. 1995.

Buckwalter, Joseph A., et al. "Exercise as a cause of osteoarthritis." In *Osteoarthritic Disorders*. Rosemont, IL: American Academy of Orthopaedic Surgeons, 1995.

Clough, John D., et al. "The new thinking on osteoarthritis." *Patient Care*, Sept. 15, 1996.

"Exercise and Arthritis." The Arthritis Foundation, 1997.

"Fitness: A Way of Life." American Physical Therapy Association, 1987.

Kovar, Pamela A., et al. "Supervised fitness walking in patients with osteoarthritis of the knee." *Annals of Internal Medicine*, vol. 116, no. 7, 1992.

Pisetsky, David S. *The Duke University Medical Center Book of Arthritis*. New York: Fawcett Columbine, 1992.

Sayce, Valerie and Ian Fraser. *Exercise for Arthritis*. Mount Vernon, NY: Consumer Reports Books, 1990.

Chapter 9.
Benzaia, Diana and Stephen Barrett. "The Misery Merchants." In *The Health Robbers: A Close Look at Quackery*

in America. Ed. Stephen Barrett and William T. Jarvis. Buffalo, NY: Prometheus Books, 1993.

Gregg, Daphna W. "Arthritis: A Harvard Health Letter Special Report." Harvard Medical School Health Publications Group, 1995.

Kantrowitz, Fred G. *Taking Control of Arthritis*. New York: HarperCollins, 1990.

Nguyen, M., et al. "Prolonged effects of 3 week therapy in a spa resort on lumbar spine, knee and hip osteoarthritis: Follow-up after 6 months. A randomized controlled trial." *British Journal of Rheumatology*, vol. 36, no. 1, 1997.

Oreizi-Esfahani, M., et al. "Traditional Chinese acupuncture is effective in the treatment of osteoarthritis of the knee." American College of Radiology Poster Session, Oct. 21, 1996.

"Questions and Answers: Glucosamine Sulfate and Chondroitin Sulfate." The Arthritis Foundation, 1997.

Sobel, Dava and Arthur C. Klein. *Arthritis: What Works*. New York: St. Martin's Press, 1989.

Strohecker, James, ed. *Alternative Medicine: The Definitive Guide*. Puyallup, WA: Future Medicine Publishing, Inc., 1994.

United States House of Representatives. Select Committee on Aging, Subcommittee on Health and Long-term Care. *Quackery: A $10 Billion Scandal*, 2 vol. Washington, D.C.: U.S. Government Printing Office, 1984.

"Unproven Remedies Fact Sheet." The Arthritis Foundation, 1997.

Chapter 10.

"Biomagnetic Treatment." The Arthritis Foundation, 1996.

"Biomatrix, Inc.'s Synvisc PMA application receives recommendation from the FDA advisory panel," Nov. 21, 1996.

Dunkin, Mary Anne. "Osteoarthritis: Undoing the damage." *Arthritis Today*, 1996.

Johannes, Laura. "Genzyme tissue repair process still in review." *Wall Street Journal*, March 7, 1997.

Moskowitz, Roland W., et. al., eds. "Cartilage growth factor (transforming growth factor-beta) in osteoarthritis." *American College of Rheumatology Hotline*, 1994.

"News Alert-Cartilage growth factor (transforming growth factor beta) in osteoarthritis." The Arthritis Foundation, 1994.

Index

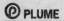 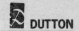